What's So Funny About®...
Heart Disease?

A Creative Approach to Coping with
Your Condition

* * *

By neurohumorist, RN,
Speaker Hall of Fame inductee
Karyn Buxman

COPYRIGHT © 2013 BY KARYN BUXMAN.

"WHAT'S SO FUNNY ABOUT® . . .?"
is a Federally Registered Trademark of Karyn Buxman.

Cover design by Poole Communications
573-221-3635 | www.PooleCommunications.com

Medical studies show that people who use humor have lower levels of stress hormones (epinephrine and norepinephrine). [1]

What's So Funny About . . .? Publishing
858-603-3133 | www.KarynBuxman.com

"If we took what we now know about laughter and bottled it, it would require FDA approval."

~ DR. LEE BERK, PSYCHONEUROIMMUNOLOGIST

DISCLAIMER

I, Karyn Buxman, RN, MSN, CSP, CPAE, LOL, FYI, CIA, PDQ, OMG, am a neurohumorist and a nurse, but not a medical doctor—or *any* kind of doctor, for that matter. For diagnosis or treatment of any medical problem (real or imagined), consult a real doctor (*not* Doctor Seuss, Doctor Dolittle or Doctor Who). The information provided in this book is designed to provide helpful information on the subjects discussed; it is not meant to be used, nor should it be used (not even once) to diagnose or treat any medical condition. The publisher and author are not responsible for any health conditions, nor are they liable for any damages or negative consequences from any treatment or action, to any person reading or following the advice contained in this book. Readers should be aware that references are provided for informational purposes only. Readers should be aware that the medical and neurological fields evolve and change. Readers should also be aware that a spoonful of sugar makes the medicine go down.

Furthermore . . . This book is not intended to be used as a flotation device. This book is not intended for dummies. Nor for idiots. This book may be harmful if swallowed. It contains a substantial amount of non-active ingredients. Not recommended for children under 12. Batteries not included. Keep away from open flame. Colors may vary, and, in time, fade.

Storage temperature: -30C (-22F) to 40C (104F). Beware of dog. Slippery when wet. You must be present to win. Use only in well-ventilated areas. Driver does not carry cash. Tag not to be removed under penalty of law. Do not read while driving or operating heavy machinery. Do not read while sleeping. Do not fold, spindle or mutilate. Do not expose to direct sunlight. Do not puncture or incinerate. Do not pass Go. Do not collect $200.

Void where prohibited by law. Or by local custom. Or by your mom. Look both ways before crossing. No smoking. No parking. No standing.. No way. Practice safe sex. But remember that practice makes perfect. And remember to send your mother a card on her birthday. Please affix proper postage. Alcohol content is less than 12% by volume. Do not drink and drive. Do not drink and read. But it's okay to drink and watch TV. Content is rated PG-13 by the Academy for Butting Into Other People's Business. Do your civic duty and vote. Do not submerge in water. Kilroy was here. Follow your doctor's recommendations. Follow your heart. Follow the Yellow Brick Road. Good grief, Charlie Brown! Use your Zip Code! Stop! Look! And Listen! Don't over-use exclamation marks!!! Don't end sentences with prepositions. Or propositions. Don't try this at home. Seek professional advice. Where's the beef? Where's Waldo? Where oh where has my little dog gone?

Authorized personnel only. An apple a day keeps the doctor away. Do not eat of the fruit of the Tree of Knowledge of Good and Evil. Objects appear smaller than they really are. Because I said so, that's why. Fragile. This side up. Handle with care. Put your right arm in, put your right arm out, put your right arm in, and shake it all about. You do the Hokey-Pokey and you turn yourself around. (That's what it's all about.)

> **Watching a sitcom can increase HDL (good cholesterol) by 26%, and decrease harmful (C-reactive) proteins by 66%.** [2]

Don't run with scissors. Don't feed the animals. Don't mix plaids with stripes. Don't have a cow, man. Don't call me Shirley. Do no evil. Do unto others as you would have them do unto you. Open sesame. Open wide. Open the pod bay doors please, Hal. Houston, we have a problem. E.T. phone home. There's no place like home. Home, home on the range. How to Make Friends and Influence People. How to Succeed in Business Without Really Trying. May cause dizziness. But—thank god, will not cause constipation.

Watch for falling rocks. Watch your P's and Q's. What, me worry? Who's on first? This offer expires after 30 days. Best if used by March 31. No trespassing. Dangerous curves ahead. Deer Xing. Merry Xmas. X marks the spot. X-rated. XOXO. Riders under 54-inches must be accompanied by an adult. 25 mpg city, 43 mpg highway. 25 or 6 to 4. The answer to life, the universe, and everything: 42. Contents may settle in shipping. Results may vary. Lather. Rinse. Repeat.

This disclaimer disclaims the disclamation of its disclaimancy. And in the end . . . The love you take is equal to the love you make.

*"Finally, here is a book that takes the evidence-based research of psychoneuroimmunology and makes it applicable for therapeutic benefit in cardiac patient care. As a nurse Karyn takes the patient on a journey of the mind-body connection with the use of the positive behavior—humor. And she tells you what humor **really** can do for you! Karyn's approach makes the reading not only humorous but also helpful. These all translate into beneficial physiology. So enjoy your journey—it is different yet therapeutic because . . . 'he who laughs lasts'!"*

~ LEE S. BERK, DrPH, MPH, FACSM, FAAIM, CHES DIRECTOR, MOLECULAR RESEARCH LAB, SCHOOL OF ALLIED HEALTH; PROFESSOR, SCHOOLS OF ALLIED HEALTH, GRADUATE & MEDICINE, LOMA LINDA UNIVERSITY

"Buxman gets to the heart of the matter as she wisely reminds us that—in addition to regular exercise, not smoking, and maintaining a low-fat diet—humor may be an important ingredient in keeping our hearts both happier and healthier."

~ ALLEN KLEIN, MA, CSP, AUTHOR OF
LEARNING TO LAUGH WHEN YOU FEEL LIKE CRYING

"What's So Funny About . . . Heart Disease? is a groundbreaking book. It focuses on using healthy humor to combat stress and promote healing. Karyn Buxman is a gifted author, speaker and nurse who shares the lighter side of the latest research in coping with this condition. This is an invaluable resource for everyone involved in the diagnosis, treatment and recovery of loved ones with heart disease."*

~ MARY KAY MORRISON, MSED, AUTHOR OF
USING HUMOR TO MAXIMIZE LIVING

"Five pages into this wonderful book, my blood pressure stabilized, my cholesterol went down, and I dropped 50 pounds!"

~ ELVIS

"I wish Karyn Buxman was my mother."

~ FREUD

*"I tip my hat to 'The **other** humorist from Hannibal, Missouri'! Karyn Buxman has written The Great American Non-Fiction Advice Book!"*

~ TWAIN

"Follow Karyn Buxman's advice! And, follow the Yellow Brick Road!"

~ GLINDA

"To be (funny), Or not to be (funny). That is the question."

~ HAMLET

Neurobiologists have proven that humor provides benefits to the cardiovascular, respiratory, immune, and musculoskeletal systems. [2]

Dedications

This book was written for many people: The people who already *know* what's so funny about heart disease, and the people who have yet to discover it. These pages were written for anyone who's ever experienced any kind of heart-related disease or incident.

This book was also written for my fellow nurses and for my colleagues in the field of therapeutic humor. You folks rock! You inspire, illuminate, imagine and create a better world every day. I am honored to be in your company.

Acknowledgments

What's so funny about heart disease? I am able to answer this question because of the support, insights and research of the following friends, colleagues, doctors and nurses.

Here's a high-five to my colleagues, mentors and friends at the Association for Applied & Therapeutic Humor. We are making the world a better place one laugh at a time. And a special shout-out to Mary Kay Morrison and the Humor Academy for giving me the shove I needed to get this project into high gear.

Kudos to Dr. Lee Berk, Dr. Michael Miller, Dr. William Fry, and the many others who have conducted the clinical research behind this book. You are making a tremendous difference in the lives of people around the planet.

Thanks to my grad school (Go Mizzou!) advisors, Virginia Bzdek, Mandy Manderino, and Sherry Mustapha. You believed in me and encouraged me to take that first step—so many years ago—in spite of the fact that most everyone else saw research into therapeutic humor as "not professional enough." Your support has been like a pebble cast into the water. I really want you to know that your influence is global in scope.

To Peter and all the regulars at the Pacific Bean Coffee Shop. Thanks for keeping me well-caffeinated during this book project. [And a special thanks for your custom "Heart Attack"—mocha with 4 (four!!) shots of espresso.]

To my colleague-turned-beloved-friend Doug Fletcher, the original publisher of the hilarous (and infamous) *Journal of Nursing Jocularity* back in the 1990s; and to my friend and mentor Dr. Vera Robinson, who, because of her pioneering work in therapeutic humor back in the 1970s, was lovingly referred to as the "Fairy Godmother of Humor."

To my advisor-and-buddy Sally and her terrific crew at Poole Communications. Thanks for making this book—and me!—look good.

A huge thank you to my editor Cindy Potts, whose talent, tenacity, and twisted sense of humor have made this entire "What's So Funny About" project a blast!

And, of course, this book would not be here were if not for my mildly-brilliant-and-oh-so-romantic-husband, Greg Godek. [*Who has more fun than you and me?*] [*Nobody!*]

Table of Contents

> *"A merry heart doeth good like a medicine."*
>
> ~ *Proverbs 17:22*

Foreword

by Michael Miller, MD

Although having a heart attack is certainly no laughing matter, changing our perception of this disease allows us to more effectively deal with the emotional burden that can slow down the healing process.

Let me begin by sharing the optimistic side of heart disease. For one, having a heart attack is no longer the death sentence it was back in the 1950s, when 1 out of every 3 heart attack patients did not survive hospitalization. During the past 60-plus years, great strides in understanding the major risk factors that contribute to heart disease, coupled with technological advances, have cut that rate to less than 5 in 100!

Equally important is the overall excellent outlook for heart disease survivors, with most being able to "get back on their feet" and return to normal, productive lives. Unfortunately, what often holds back the recovery process among survivors of heart attacks or open-heart surgery is the emotional consequences that can include depression, a lost sense of invincibility and increased feelings of inadequacy. While several books have been written about some of these concerns, none have integrated them in a way that is especially appealing to healthcare providers and patients alike . . . until now.

What's So Funny About . . . Heart Disease? represents the logical sequel to Karyn Buxman's critically acclaimed book *What's So Funny About . . . Diabetes?* For more than a quarter century, Karyn has been a powerful voice in applied and therapeutic humor, engaging her audiences worldwide with her keen sense of humor, wit and vast medical knowledge. There are many outstanding comedians and healthcare professionals, but it is the very "rare bird" who can find the lighter side to serious diseases in a thoughtful manner that is also very instructive to patients. Karyn has that gift.

Having also been in the medical field for more than a quarter century, with research experience in the field of laughter and cardiovascular medicine, I anticipate that *What's So Funny About . . . Heart Disease?* will generate a great deal of enthusiasm because of the many, many new and useful tips that Karyn provides. I believe that it will make a difference in the lives of many patients with heart disease and help them to live active, healthy and happy lives. Karyn has made a difference in *my* life. And I know that *my* patients will benefit, too!

MICHAEL MILLER, MD, FACC, FAHA

PROFESSOR OF MEDICINE, UNIVERSITY OF MARYLAND SCHOOL OF MEDICINE

DIRECTOR, CENTER FOR PREVENTIVE CARDIOLOGY, UNIVERSITY OF MARYLAND MEDICAL CENTER, BALTIMORE, MARYLAND

"What's the worst time

to have a heart attack?

When you're playing charades!"

~ KARYN BUXMAN, NEUROHUMORIST

Introduction

"Funny? . . . You think I'm *funny*? I'll tell you what—You're right. I *am* funny. As funny as a *heart attack!*"

These lines from a tough guy in a 1940s gangster movie bring us to the first question . . . What, exactly, *is* funny about heart disease? Whether you've had a heart attack, coronary artery disease, a faulty valve, a congenital heart condition, or any of the dozen other conditions that come under the umbrella of "heart disease," you might be wondering exactly that.

The truth is, heart disease is no joke. However, the situations that arise as a result of your condition can be material for an entire stand-up comedy routine. (See "David Letterman" on page 139!)

It sure doesn't *seem* like there's much that's funny about heart disease. But you might be surprised. A lot of adult humor comes from pain and discomfort—maybe it's our own, maybe it's somebody else's. And if there's one thing that heart disease can do, it's deliver pain and discomfort.

*"Tragedy is when I cut my finger.
Comedy is when you
walk into an open sewer and die."*
~ MEL BROOKS

Let's look at what makes us laugh. Usually, we're not doubled over in hysterics over our great hair, or fabulous golf game, or super-sexy figure. We don't laugh because we have more money than Donald Trump [and he's *definitely* not having a good hair day, but I digress…]. When we laugh, we laugh about the things that make us crazy. And let's face it, if you have heart disease, you've got more than your fair share of crazy-making things in your life!

Heart disease is a fabulous motivator. You may have been laid-back and easygoing about your health and fitness in the past, but find that now you're as serious as a heart attack about them. It soon becomes clear that *you need to arm yourself with all the tools at your disposal in order to become the healthiest person that you can be.*

Living a healthy life with heart disease can be tough. There's a lot involved. It helps tremendously to have a large repertoire of skills. You want a full toolbox of resources to help you navigate the many life changes that come with heart disease.

Humor is a tool in that toolbox. A powerful tool,

but not the *only* tool . . . Humor isn't the end-all-be-all of treatments. No responsible healthcare professional would try to convince you otherwise. What the enlightened healthcare professionals *will* tell you is that *humor has a powerful role to play in your heart health routine.* It is a great tool to complement and enhance all of the other efforts you're already making. All of those positive changes to your diet, the new exercise routine, and your commitment to stop stressing-out, all work better and are easier to stick to when you use humor.

Humor isn't just for comedians! Many people worry that they're not "funny enough" to benefit from the healing power of humor. They ask me, "Can you teach me to be funny?" And if push came to shove, I could absolutely teach them a short comedy bit that might serve their purposes every so often. But it's not about *being* funny as much as it is about *seeing* funny.

If you can "*see* funny," the "*be* funny" will fall into place.

Everyone has a sense of humor [although you might need the Hubble Space Telescope to find it in some people!]. The fact that you've picked-up and are reading this book means the chances are even better that yours is a *good, positive* sense of humor. By understanding what humor is and how it works, you can put that sense of humor to work for you.

But wait . . . there's *more!* When you start using humor proactively as part of your heart health routine, you're going to find that humor helps you in a lot of *other* areas of your life. That's because humor has far-reaching *physiological* benefits, *psychological* benefits, and *social* benefits. Humor makes getting along with other people much easier. Humor is also a social lubricant—it helps strengthen relationships and build rapport; and the more you use humor, the easier it becomes!

There may be another link between humor and heart disease. As a person with heart disease, you're in the company of some very funny folks. George Carlin, Rosie O'Donnell, Robin Williams, Elizabeth Banks, Lewis Grizzard, Red Buttons, Peter Sellers, Regis Philbin and David Letterman have all dealt with heart disease—and used the experiences in some of their funniest material! (Heart disease doesn't necessarily *make* you funny, but it sure didn't get in the way of the success of these folks!)

So fasten your seatbelt, put your tray table in the upright and locked position, and let's go!

YOURS IN LAUGHTER!

KARYN BUXMAN, RN, MSN, CSP, CPAE, NEUROHUMORIST

RN: REGISTERED NURSE

MSN: MASTERS DEGREE IN MENTAL HEALTH NURSING

CSP: CERTIFIED SPEAKING PROFESSIONAL

CPAE: THE SPEAKER HALL OF FAME (THE OSCARS OF THE SPEAKING PROFESSION)

NEUROHUMORIST: ONE WHO RESEARCHES THE NEUROBIOLOGY AND PSYCHOLOGY OF HUMOR, AND THEN TRANSLATES CUTTING-EDGE FINDINGS INTO PRACTICAL IDEAS FOR THE LAYPERSON.

"Laughter is medicine to the weary bones."

~ CARL SANDBURG

"When you have something like heart surgery, you appreciate the simple things in life — like breathing."

~ ROBIN WILLIAMS

Chapter 1

What's NOT So Funny About Heart Disease?

Having heart disease puts you in one of the world's largest clubs.[1] Last year, 1.2 million people in the U.S. had a new or recurrent cardiac event.[2] That's one person every 25 seconds—two a minute!

While club membership is growing fast, no one really *wants* their membership. Heart disease is the #1 killer of women and men.[3] [Well, there's *one* thing the two genders have in common!]

I know, I know—it's a laugh-a-minute here. But it's important that we know and acknowledge that heart disease is a really serious condition. Being diagnosed is life-changing. It's overwhelming, even terrifying, to contemplate the new level of worry and responsibility that comes when the doctor says, "I have some news for you. You'd better sit down."

So before we start discovering the *funny* side of heart disease, I'm going to come right out and say that having heart disease is no joke. Sticking to your heart health regimen of diet, exercise, and stress reduction matters a lot! Failing to take your disease seriously can have some nasty—if not deadly—consequences.

For example, did you know . . . ?

- Having a heart attack dramatically increases the likelihood you'll have *another* heart attack. Within a year, approximately 1 in 10 people *will* experience a second heart attack—especially if that 1 in 10 doesn't make the necessary lifestyle changes. (After a year, the risk drops to about 1 in 30.) [3]

- Heart disease is swell—or more correctly, it can *make* you swell! Edema and other conditions characterized by the painful retention of fluids are all exacerbated by heart disease. [4, 6]

- Heart disease can take your breath away. [5, 6] Shortness of breath is a real SOB. [That is, "Short Of Breath"!]

- You've never felt so tired. Extreme fatigue, exhaustion, and not having enough energy to do everything you want to do in a day are all tied to your heart health. If your heart isn't pumping that oxygenated blood throughout your body, you're going to feel it. [5, 6]

- Numbness, pain and stroke-like symptoms are more common in cardiac patients who don't follow their heart health regimen. [6]

- Heart disease affects your emotional and mental health. Depression, anxiety and extreme mood swings are common aftereffects of a cardiac event. [7]

If all that weren't bad enough, heart disease can even make us get older faster! [Hold on, I think that last sentence just gave *me* a heart attack!] According to a recent study reported in *Circulation: Journal of the American Heart Association*, there is a likely connection between heart disease and how quickly our brains age. [8] All of our brains get smaller as we age [oh, why couldn't it be *waistlines* that shrink as we age??] but it's those of us whose hearts have the most

> **Heart disease is the leading cause of death in America.** [8]

difficulty pumping adequate amounts of blood to the brain that see the shrinkage happen fastest. This has an obvious impact on our ability to think, feel, and function.

Okay, so having heart disease is not fun or humorous. I'm not trying to make light of this serious condition. But while heart disease itself is *not* funny, your experiences and your life *can* be funny.

The premise of this book [borne out by scientific research conducted by real researchers and academics with all kinds of impressive letters after their names—and who wear white lab coats!] is that humor has many practical benefits for heart disease patients. You can use laughter to enhance the lifestyle changes you're making, resulting in a longer, happier life.

You *can* make a difference in your health—so let's get going!

"Laughter is the most inexpensive and most effective wonder drug."

~ BERTRAND RUSSELL

"There ain't much fun in medicine — but there's a heck of a lot of medicine in fun."

~ JOSH BILLINGS

Chapter 2

What Humor Can Do for You

Now it's time for some GOOD news! While we've known since Biblical times that laughter makes us feel better—"A merry heart doeth good like a medicine." (Proverbs 17:22)—science is finally starting to prove it!

In Medieval times it was thought that if the body's fluids (known then as "umors") were in balance, one was of good temperament—or healthy. That's where the phrase "having a good sense of humor" came from. The umors were yellow bile, black bile, blood, and lymph.

Throughout the Middle Ages, the practice of medicine was more art than science. And as art goes—well, let's just say you should be glad you didn't live back in the Days of Yore! The following is from a *Saturday Night Live* skit, with comedian Steve Martin playing Theodoric of York, a doctor/barber:

> *"You know, medicine is not an exact science,*
> *but we are learning all the time.*
> *Why, just fifty years ago, they thought a disease*
> *like your daughter's*
> *was caused by demonic possession or witchcraft.*
> *But nowadays we know that Isabelle is suffering from an*
> *imbalance of bodily humors,*
> *perhaps caused by a toad or a small dwarf*
> *living in her stomach."* [10]

We now know that umor, or humor, isn't a body fluid at all. [And it's pretty rare indeed to find a toad or small dwarf living in anyone's stomach.] But I digress . . .

So, if humor isn't a body fluid—exactly what *is* it? Here's the most *concise* definition . . .

> *"Humor is whatever people find funny."*
>
> ~ Elaine Pasquali

Hmmm . . . This may the most *concise* definition—but is it the most *insightful* definition?

———————

How about a *psychoanalyst's* view? Sigmund Freud's definition is . . .

> *"Humor is a coping mechanism*
> *that allows persons to reduce tension and anxiety*
> *by expressing obscene or hostile impulses*
> *in a socially acceptable manner."*

That's rather intense, isn't it?! It certainly contains some truth. But is it really helpful?? Perhaps not.

———————

How about a *comedian's* opinion? Groucho Marx said . . .

> *"Humor is reason gone mad."*

Hmmm . . . Short is good. Funny is good. But perhaps this is a little *too* pithy.

———————

How about an *educator's* thoughts? Joel Goodman, founder of The HUMORProject, weighs in with . . .

"Humor is a childlike perspective
in an otherwise serious adult reality."

Hmmm . . . I like this one!

And how about a *psychologist's* point-of-view? One therapist, Steve Sultanoff, Ph.D. said . . .

*"Humor is the **intellectual** mindset that is expressed*
*through the **emotional** feelings of mirth*
*and the **physical** expression of laughter."*

Hmmm . . . I like this one, too! It links the intellectual, emotional and physical modalities with the three elements that comprise humor: Mindset, mirth and laughter.

And finally, perhaps we should consider a defintion from a *neurohumorist:*

"Humor is a feeling of delight, wonder or release—
that comes from surprise, perspective or insight."

Oh, wait! That's *my* definition of humor. [I'm rather partial to it, but I won't insist! I've given you six definitions, so you you can choose the one that works best for you, or mix-and-match them to create your *own* definition of humor.]

———

Delight. Wonder. Release. I love the idea of looking at life through the eyes of a child; they have such a sense of fun and playfulness [which we seem to lose as we get older, more serious, and more "professional"]. And perspective is the underpinning of all reframing—our ability to *see* funny, and ultimately our ability to just be happier.

True story . . . from the Karyn Buxman Archives:

> It was eight o'clock on a Monday morning. In my haste to get myself ready for the work day, I'd temporarily forgotten about my seven-year-old son. A rhythmic thumping noise coming from upstairs brought him back to mind.
>
> A mom-on-a-mission, I ran up the stairs. As I approached Adam's room I could feel the *Whomp! Whomp! Whomp!* vibrating through the walls.
>
> What in the world—?!" I wondered.
>
> I opened his door and saw Adam—wearing nothing but his underwear and a big smile . . . jumping up and down on his bed . . .

. . . singing and dancing . . . swinging his shirt over and around his head . . . with enthusiastic kicks accenting the beat.

"What do you think you're doing, young man?" I demanded.

Adam stopped mid-jump, grinned a huge grin, and with the wisdom of Yoda, said, "Don't-ya-think-getting-dressed-in-the-morning-oughta-be-more-*fun*, Mom?!"

Let's think about this . . . What if *getting dressed* in the morning *could* be more fun? What if *getting up in the morning* could be more fun? What if *going to work* could be more fun?! By playing with our perspective, we can create a happier experience—for ourselves, for our friends, and for our families.

———

Humor is definitely a bit of a paradox. [Not to be confused with a pair-of-ducks. (Sometimes I quack myself up!)]

Humor can come from surprise. Humor can come from "derailment"—that sudden unexpected twist that makes a good joke work so well.

Humor can come from pure delight. (Watch young children for example. Older folks don't experience nearly as much pure delight in living and discovering the world around them.)

And, believe it or not, sometimes humor and laughter can come from pain and discomfort. (See: Banana peel; most practical jokes; or the Wiley Coyote dropping an anvil on his own head, in the pursuit of the Road Runner.)

How *important* is humor? Consider this:

"The old saying that 'laughter is the best medicine,' definitely appears to be true when it comes to protecting your heart," says Michael Miller, M.D., Director of the Center for Preventive Cardiology at the University of Maryland Medical Center and a professor of medicine at the University of Maryland School of Medicine. *"The ability to laugh—either naturally or as a learned behavior—may have important implications in societies*

In 2010, coronary heart disease alone cost the U.S. about $108 billion. [4]

such as the U.S. where heart disease remains the number one killer . . . We know that exercising, not smoking, and eating foods low in saturated fat will reduce the risk of heart disease. Perhaps regular, hearty laughter should be added to the list." [3]

There has been a lot of serious research into what makes us laugh—and what laughter does for us. These studies come from part of a broader field of research called psychoneuroimmunology. What?? That's psych-neuro-immunology (psycho = mind; neuro = nervous system; immunology = immune system)—which is sometimes referred to as the mind-body connection. Some experts throw in the endocrine system, too, making this the study of "psychoneuroimmunoendocrinology." [Frankly, I think these scientists are frustrated Scrabble players.] For simplicity [and sanity], I'll refer to this as PNI from here on out.

The rest of this chapter presents the highlights of that research, particularly as it pertains to people with heart disease or diabetes. (Having diabetes puts you at increased risk for heart disease.)[4]

What Humor Can Do for Your *Body*

Humor and laughter have many positive effects on your body. PNI is a maturing field, and recent studies are proving that laughter provides positive benefits to nearly every body system: Cardiovascular, respiratory, immune, and musculo-skeletal, just to name a few.[5, 6] But some of these effects are going to be of more interest to you than others.

"The old man laughed loud and joyously, shook up the details of his anatomy from head to foot, and ended by saying such a laugh was money in a man's pocket, because it cut down the doctor's bills like everything."

~ MARK TWAIN

Let's Get to The Heart of The Matter

Humor has been shown to help some people reduce their *bad* cholesterol (LDL) while increasing their *good* cholesterol (HDL). In a study conducted by psychoneuroimmunologist Dr. Lee Berk, and his colleague, Dr. Stanley Tan, diabetic patients spent half an hour a day watching movies or sitcoms that they found humorous. As a result, their levels of HDL (the good cholesterol) increased by 26%, while harmful C-reactive proteins declined by 66%. [7] When was the last time you heard that watching TV could actually make you healthier? [So now I can admit to my "Scooby-Doo" habit.]

And here's the connection between diabetics and heart patients: Reducing cholesterol is Job Number One if you have heart disease. (It's very likely that your doctor has prescribed medication to control or reduce your cholesterol levels.) So by proactively practicing more humor and laughter, you can reduce your risk for further complications of cardiovascular disease. Reducing cholesterol is one example of how humor can do more than make you *feel* better: Humor can help you *be* better!

Lower Your Inflammation

Budgets, deadlines, timelines, crazy relatives, irritable spouses, traffic jams . . . For many of us a straight jacket may be nearer than we think! And whether the source of stress is at work or at home, the results on our health can be costly. According to Dr. Lee Berk, stress exacerbates inflammation in our bodies. This is one of the reasons plaque builds up in our blood vessels; it is the body's attempt to heal the inflammation on the lining of our arteries. The more inflammation, the more plaque accumulates. And a buildup of plaque can cause blockage in our blood vessels, which leads to high blood pressure, heart attacks or strokes.

Studies have shown that participants who used humor and laughter had lower levels of stress hormones (such as epi-

> *The average human heart beats 100,000 times a day. That's 2.5 billion beats in an average lifetime!* [7]

nephrine and norepinephrine), as well as lower levels of markers for inflammation (C-reactive proteins and cytokines) which lead to atherosclerosis and cardiovascular disease.[8] Okay. In layman's terms, this means lifestyle choices—like diet, exercise *and* humor—can have a significant positive impact on your heart health.

Decrease Your Blood Pressure

Enjoying laughter can help lower your blood pressure. In a study conducted by the Osaka University Graduate School of Medicine, in Japan, 90 men and women between the ages of 40 and 74 participated in hour-long music or laughter sessions every other week. After three months, the average systolic blood pressure had dropped by 6 mmHg for men and 5 mmHg for women. There were also short-term drops in blood pressure that were apparent immediately after the laughter sessions.

What does this mean? Dr. Michael Miller, a preventative cardiologist, says that this result is equivalent to adopting a low-salt diet, losing ten pounds, or taking a prescription medication.[9] Just imagine how great you'll feel when you're doing *all* of these things—*and* laughing!

Increase Your Circulation

Humor can help you increase your circulation. That's great news if you're suffering from the numb fingers, tingling pain, or aches in your extremities so often associated with heart disease. All of these complaints have their origin in decreased circulation.

Back in 1977, Dr. William Fry, one of the pioneers researching the relationship between heart health and laughter, began proving that hearty laughter has a positive impact on circulation rates.[10, 11] So go ahead and laugh. You'll do more than just have fun, you'll experience some of the groundbreaking discoveries of Dr. Fry. You'll be getting an increased supply of freshly oxygenated blood moving throughout your body. Better circulation results in less numbness and extremity pain, and faster healing from minor nicks, scrapes and wounds. It is also great news for your brain, your energy levels, and your overall health!

Blood Sugar (Glucose) Control

"Why should I worry about blood sugar? I don't have diabetes!"

That's what you may be asking. But trust me, blood sugar (or glucose) control should be of interest to you. This is especially true if your doctor has prescribed statins for your condition. Surprisingly, recent studies have indicated that long-term statin use may be a contributing factor in the development of Type 2 diabetes.[12] The right lifestyle choices can help minimize that risk.

So bring on the humor! Humor can help lower the increase in blood sugar you experience after eating a meal. Another study from Japan showed that people who watched a brief comedy show after eating had lower glucose values than those who did not see the program.[13, 14] Pretty sweet!

Studies show that laughing lowers your levels of the stress hormones cortisol and adrenaline. Cortisol increases insulin resistance, while adrenaline tells your liver to pump more glucose into your blood.[15] The combined effect can be a lasting reduction in blood glucose levels. In other words, laughter can probably help lower your blood glucose and keep it down for quite a while!

Improve Your Vasuclar Health

Remember Dr. Miller? He's the one who led an exciting study at the University of Maryland which *shows for the first time that laughter is linked to the healthy function of blood vessels.* Laughter appears to cause the tissue that forms the inner lining of blood vessels (the endothelium) to dilate, or expand, in order to increase blood flow.[16]

"We know it works!" he told me. There's an apparent relationship between mental stress and vasoconstriction—the narrowing, or tightening, of your blood vessels. We don't want our blood vessels tight and constricted. We want them to be wide open, flexible and healthy highways for the transport of oxygenated blood. "The endothelium is one of the most basic cardiac mechanisms," explains Dr. Miller. "The fact that it is highly responsive to robust laughter means we have a real story here. And there's no downside to laughter!" [And how many procedures

> *Recent studies show that people who actively use humor and laughter have lower levels of markers for inflammation (C-reactive proteins and cytokines) which lead to atheroclerosis and cardiovascular disease.* [1]

or medicines do you know of that don't have any neg-ative side effects?!]

Pain Management

Remember when you were a teenager and you thought nothing could hurt worse than your broken heart? It turns out that you were wrong. Heart disease has its own suite of associated aches and pains, mak-ing pain management a new part of your daily routine.

Laughter lowers blood pressure and reduces anxi-ety and inflammation. This helps relieve pain through-out the body.[8] [Pain *outside* your body is beyond our scope of practice—sorry! Our humor seems to be of little help in fighting crime or global warming.]

The Ohio State University Medical Center pro-vides their patients with a handout detailing the value of humor in pain management. By providing a distrac-tion, humor shifts your focus away from the pain and onto whatever you're laughing at. It doesn't *eliminate* the pain, but it helps you *deal with it* more effectively. Humor reduces the prominent position pain plays in your day.

What Humor Can Do for Your *Emotions*

Now let's talk about the *psychological* benefits of humor. And there are lots of them!

Some of these benefits are *immediate* benefits. Laughter works fast! It makes you feel good. You'll feel your mood lifting, and it gets much easier to maintain a positive outlook. [6, 17, 18]

But wait—there's more! Humor helps fight heart disease by providing you with *long-term* benefits. Laugh today, and you can feel better tomorrow, too! Here's how . . .

Provides an Outlet for Anger

If you ask me, one of humanity's greatest inventions is language. We use the power of words to communicate so many feelings—love, fear, excitement, passion. Humor is a special type of communication, used for specific situations.

> *"Language was created to communicate. Humor was created to complain."*
>
> ~ KARYN BUXMAN

Dealing with a chronic condition such as heart disease can trigger anger. There's anger that this has happened at all, and that it's happened to YOU, and that your life is disrupted and permanently changed. Anger is an extremely common response to heart disease.

Humor is a wonderful way to help process and transform anger. [6, 19] Many comedians assert that much of their best material comes out of the times in their lives when they were angriest. [We did not ask Jon Stewart. We assume *his* best material comes out of Washington!] And while people will run like the building is on fire when a complainer approaches, humor can be a socially acceptable—even enjoyable—way for people to vent.

Part of having a chronic condition—*any* chronic condition—is that you're going to be frustrated, you're going to be angry, and you're going to have moments when you're filled with rage. It's unrealistic to think that embracing humor as a coping strategy is going to eliminate all of those feelings.

In fact, eliminating those feelings isn't even the point. Trying to ignore or stifle feelings of anger and frustration that come with heart disease just doesn't work. Repressing your emotions can make things even worse!

Humor redirects anger, instead of avoiding or denying it. This redirection can defuse a lot of rage, bringing with it a sense of calm, relief and a fresh perspective. The underlying circumstances that made us

angry still exist, but after we've laughed we're better prepared to address those circumstances.

*"It is impossible for you to be angry and laugh at the
same time. Anger and laughter are mutually exclusive
and you have the power to choose either."*

~ Wayne Dyer

It feels good to laugh at problems, if only for a
moment. This doesn't mean closing our eyes to reality.
Instead, laughter allows us to reframe the issue and look
at it anew. Sometimes a change in perspective presents
the information we need in order to move past the anger.

Reduces Stress

Humor is a powerful tool for stress reduction.[19, 20]
You may have heard a thing or two about the need for
stress reduction since your cardiac event. [Hey, you Type
A's over there in the corner: This section is for *you*!]
Many of you believe that you thrive in high-stress, high-
tension environments. You may happen to have skills
that allow you to thrive in high-stress situations when
other people wouldn't be able to function at all. On the

surface, it looks great! But under the surface, your heart and cardiovascular system are suffering, and eventually, something is going to blow. You'll meet plenty of fellow successful Type A people at cardiac rehab!

Learning how to effectively manage stress is an integral part of your heart health routine. The simple fact that you *have* heart disease is stressful . . . and on top of *that*, managing a new heart health routine in addition to all your other professional, family, and community responsibilities is pretty stressful, too!

Humor is recognized by healthcare professionals as a healthy coping mechanism. [5, 6, 19, 20] It's perfect for stress management. Laughing makes us feel good. Sure—eating, drinking and smoking to excess may feel good temporarily, but these behaviors can make you sicker, and even kill you, in the long-run. Humor relieves anxiety and tension, provides a healthy escape from reality, and lightens heaviness related to those aspects of heart disease that really weigh you down.

A Time for Mirth, a Time to Mourn

There are things we tend not to talk about, and one of those things is the very real fact that heart disease takes things away from us. We lose, when we have a heart attack. The shadow of further heart trouble, up to and including a second or third heart attack, can strip the joy from our days. We worry if we'll ever have a fear-free day. We may not be able to do everything we used to do, in the way we'd like to do it. It's hard to skip those bacon-double-cheeseburgers—especially when they're served with a double order of double-fried French Fries.

These losses are real. All of them, from the serious to the silly. We need a time to grieve and mourn what we've lost.   Realize that it's not at all uncommon ["medical speak" for "This happens to everyone!"] for people who have just learned that "What's wrong with me?" isn't just the flu or being over-tired or a simple psychiatric breakdown, but is, instead, a disease that will be with them for the rest of their lives. Experiencing a profound sense of loss is completely normal in this situation.

After his heart surgery, Lewis Grizzard wrote, "It is still too early to tell what profound effects this experience will have on me. I think I am better for it, obviously physically and probably otherwise, but I would not recommend it as a way of making improvements on one's self until all other avenues, such as seeing a chiropractor or joining a couple of religious movements, have been exhausted."[21]

But like Grizzard, you get no choice in the matter.

Not now. If you think back, you might notice that at no time did someone take you aside and say, "Hey, buddy, want to have a heart attack? What about COPD? I've got a little arrhythmia here that no one can resist—your heart will be moving like a Mexican jumping bean before you count to three!" You're stuck with the diagnosis you've been given. At this point in life, you don't get to choose.

One study produced significant decreases in blood pressure among people who had participated in bi-weekly "laughter sessions." [1]

So we have a situation where we don't like the circumstances we're in. We didn't even get to make a choice about whether we want these circumstances in our life. This is a pretty serious thing here, and it's sad. There will be times you'll want to mourn this loss. There's no need to feel ashamed, pressured, or silly about this. It's a natural part of the process. It happens to everyone.

It's also—believe-it-or-not—one of the best sources of humor in the world. I'd like to draw your attention to Rodney Dangerfield for a moment. Love him or hate him, you've got to respect the fact that he's built an entire career out of the fact that he gets, well, no respect. Getting no respect is not something

Rodney chose, nor is it something he wanted. [At least not at first. Eventually it started working for him.] But he took that concept and used it to build a life of laughter. When we are done mourning, we can do the same.

Be aware that mourning isn't an all-or-nothing deal. It happens. Grief comes and goes. You can be feeling fine one minute, and then something happens that throws you right back into a discouraged mood. The thing to do is to mourn when you need to mourn, and then let it go and move on. Think of mourning as an exercise your psyche must go through periodically in order to keep in shape. It's necessary, but you don't have to stay in that mode all of the time.

And last but not least, Steve Wilson, founder of World Laughter Tour, has this to say: "Even if there were no evidence whatsoever that laughter changed a thing in your physiology—I want a life filled with laughter and humor. Laughter is its own reward, darn it. It feels good! Humor helps me see the world in better balance. Good natured laughter connects me to others, and that feels great. And, a life absent of laughter and humor is too dreadful to contemplate."[22] [Now there's somebody who really *gets it*!]

What Humor Can Do for You *Socially*

Laugh and the World Laughs with You

A diagnosis of heart disease can result in isolation. Even though heart disease isn't contagious, there are people who act as if it was. You may notice family and friends staying away. Some people can't handle the emotional pressure of knowing you've had a heart attack; others are worried that you'll keel over right in front of them.

There are other ways that heart disease can strain your relationships. There's nothing like a cardiac event to bring out the inner nutritionist in some people. They'll watch every bite you eat, sure that if they can steer you from the fat-filled Oreos to the pure and shining path of heart-healthy oatmeal, you'll live forever. This is the type of thing that can really strain a relationship. At a minimum, you might want to avoid eating with these folks. In other instances, it becomes tempting not to see them at all. Ever.

Humor is an effective way to combat social isolation.[6, 19, 20] You can use humor to directly address some of the issues that crop up in your relationships. For example, if a friend wants to act like she's your mother and take charge of your daily lunch choices, treat her like she *is* your mother—and ask her for twenty bucks!

"Laughter is the shortest distance between two people."

~ VICTOR BORGE

Humor has been found to strengthen existing relationships [which is good if you *like* the people you know!]. Regular use of humor is thought to make us more attractive to other people, which can increase your social circle and your base of support [this is good news if you *don't* like the people you currently know].

Heart disease does have one positive social aspect. You're going to meet a lot of people. From the friendly crew at the Emergency Room to your Cardiologist and his or her team, the folks at the Cardiac Rehab center, the staff at the gym, the produce guy at the local grocery store . . . the list is endless. And, as you live with heart disease, it is inevitable that you will meet other people who have heart disease.

Some of these people have just found out they have heart disease. Remember how scared you were when you were first diagnosed? Chances are these folks feel the same way. This is your chance to effect some positive change in the world, and in their lives.

These new heart disease patients tend to have lots of questions. Luckily, there are lots of people out there who can teach them about counting carbs and the wonders of exercise.

My suggestion is to let someone *else* handle that clinical and boring stuff. You can have some real fun instead by teaching the newbies about the value of humor. Share some of your favorite funny stories. Let's say you tell the tale of the time your wayward grandson stole your nitro—he wanted to blow up the school and miss his math exam. You'll be doing more than making people laugh. You're sharing your own heart disease experiences, letting other people know that these things happen, and that they're survivable. There's a lot of comfort delivered with those chuckles. You'll be leading by example, and removing some of the fear the 'new guy' may be feeling. Let them know it's okay to laugh.

"There's real benefit in the support that our patients get from each other," says Mary Kaye Bushmeyer, RN who worked for many years as Senior Director of Cardiac Services. "They work out together, they talk together, they support each other through ups and downs, but most importantly, they laugh together."

Levels the Playing Field

Humor helps us connect. This is true, even in those awkward moments when you think you have nothing in common with the people who surround you. It doesn't matter what race you are, what gender or what religion you are, or how much money you make [or don't make]. If something's funny, people laugh.

Social scientists say that laughter has the power to reduce hierarchies.[23] That means we're all on the same level when we laugh. This makes it easier for people from all different types of life circumstances to connect with each other. When we can laugh together, communication becomes easier. Whether it's doctor/patient, boss/worker, parent/child, or some other relationship, when people are enjoying true mirthful laughter, they're connecting on a one-to-one basis.

Norman Cousins, who did so much groundbreaking work on the connection between humor and healing, was in the hospital after a coronary event. He had a hard time getting on that level playing field with his nurse, who insisted on talking to him in "We" language.

You know the type. She's the nurse who would give him the urinal cup, and say, "We shall fill it up now."

Mr. Cousins, ever polite, would say, "You do it first."

One day he filled the urinal cup with his favorite apple juice. When the nurse came to pick it up, she held it up and said, "It has an unusual color today." That's when Mr. Cousins grabbed the cup and drank it down, exclaiming, "Maybe the second time around it can become clearer!" [24]

You'd better believe that nurse never saw the mischievous Mr. Cousins as just a patient again. At that point, he became a very memorable person in her eyes!

What Humor Can Do for Your *Communications*

Gets Your Message Across

One of the cool things about humor is that it makes it easier for us to communicate. [6] Teachers, preachers, speakers, and politicians all agree: If you want to get someone listening, get them laughing. People enjoy laughing. When you've provided them with something humorous to enjoy, they're more likely to listen to the rest of what you have to say in the hopes that they'll get to laugh again.

That's important information to have if you find yourself in a situation where you really need someone to listen to you. You may feel uncomfortable or ill at ease even bringing the topic up. That's when humor shines.

"Ever since I had my heart attack, my wife acts like I'm made out of glass," explains Simon. "I can't do anything without her hovering around. Stupid things. I can't take the trash out—and this is the woman who's been telling me to take the trash out since 1984!" Simon shook his head. "I understand that she's scared. But enough is enough. Finally, one day I was headed to use the bathroom, and she was all, "Where are you going?" So I asked her to come along and give me a hand. It shocked her, and it made her laugh, and finally, we got to where we could talk about what I could and couldn't do."

Humor can serve as a safety net for difficult con versations. Simon needed his wife to back off with the over-the-top concern without minimizing her very real worry and anxiety. Using a joke that brought the situation into an absurd spotlight—obviously a grown man can use the bathroom on his own!—provided the opening needed to address the larger issue.

Using humor lets you bring up serious subjects in a lighthearted manner. It's a way to test the waters with your audience. If they respond well to the humor, it becomes easier to move the conversation forward and address larger issues. Even humor that doesn't necessarily *work* can also spark meaningful, much-needed conversations. Humor can open the door to important communication, whether it's a doctor, nurse, family member or friend.

"Many a true word is spoken in jest."
~ ENGLISH PROVERB

On the other hand, there are times when humor can get it the way. If you have a serious concern, making jokes about it with your doctor or nurse may open the door for conversation. Then again, they may miss the cue entirely. It's not a good idea to use humor to evade a serious issue that may affect your health. You can't count on your medical team to be mind readers. If you have a concern, worry or question, ask them directly. Don't wait for them to bring the issue up. [And don't wait for the perfect straight line that will allow you to launch into your comedy bit.]

"Humor by CHANCE can be beneficial, but humor by CHOICE creates amazing, life-changing results."

~ KARYN BUXMAN, NEUROHUMORIST

Chapter 3

Humor: The Good, the Bad and the Ugly

Laughing WITH or Laughing *AT?*

Laugh, and the world laughs with you—but not everyone will laugh at everything. There are many types of humor, and there are many types of people. It may be that the joke that makes you laugh so hard you wet your pants leaves your best friend asking, "What's so funny about *that?*" Humor is not one size fits all!

Some types of humor are healthier than others. There is humor that makes you feel really good, upbeat and ready to take on the world. And then there is humor that, while you may laugh, leaves you feeling angry, upset, dismissed or minimized—in other words, really, really bad.

Sarcasm is a type of humor that can leave some of us laughing and others upset. When we look at word origins, we discover that the root word of sarcasm actually means "to tear the flesh". [Ouch!] And if you've ever been sniped with a sarcastic remark, you may feel like you were missing a bit of hide.

Does that mean we have to pass on the sarcasm? No, but it does mean that we need to be mindful of who and what we're sarcastic about. Humor that hurts others in the long-run doesn't help you.

Understanding the Types of Humor

Humor comes in a number of flavors [all of which are low-fat, low-calorie, and approved for your diet!]. There's constructive humor—the light, upbeat type of humor that builds people up. [A side benefit is that it builds you up, too!] And then there's destructive humor, which is a more negative type of humor, where we find the laughs at other people's expense. Wise to avoid!

People sometimes worry about their ability to tell the two types of humor apart. Taken to extremes, this concern keeps people from using humor at all, for fear they may offend someone. However, most of us have the social skills and insights that make telling constructive humor and destructive humor apart relatively easy. Relax! It's not as hard as you might think.

If you find yourself thinking, "I'm going to hell for joking about this," it's likely negative humor. If you would feel ashamed if someone you respected—a parent, boss, friend—heard the joke, it's likely negative humor. If someone you didn't like told you the joke you were just telling, would you find yourself offended and incensed? Negative humor.

It's a matter of laughing *with* someone rather than laughing *at* someone. It's always healthier to laugh *with* others than to laugh *at* them. Healthy humor builds the bonds between people.

One type of humor that usually works well is self-deprecating humor—making fun of yourself. No one will be offended, and it will actually show people that your self-esteem is strong enough to withstand being teased. Self-deprecating humor can actually increase other people's opinion of you!

A Word (or 872) about "Sick Humor"

"The heart attack didn't kill me off, so now she's using the treadmill to do it." Pete M. nodded toward his wife Lily, who accompanies her husband to the cardiac rehab center. "She wants to make sure she gets that life insurance money while she's still young enough to spend it!"

Lily, who is 81, is not amused by Pete's joke. She's hardly the first spouse to hear this kind of kidding—morbid and "sick" jokes are a very common way for people to deal with the stress, tension, and anxiety that come with heart disease.

In fact, anyone who deals with traumatic situations is likely to count on some type of "sick humor" to help them keep their balance amid difficult situations. For example, soldiers, policemen, firemen and health-care workers all have their own style of "sick humor" that actually helps them get by, and also bonds them to one another.

It's a special brand of humor that is not meant for outsiders. And that's logical, because if you've never experienced what they have, you're not really a member of their "tribe." Any kind of humor that makes you laugh, whether it's sick or not, is going to relieve your stress. It may not, however, do much for the stress of the people around you. Those who share your pain and experiences will "get it." Those that don't, won't.

That's important to keep in mind when you're joking with spouses, partners and loved ones. They love you, but if they haven't had a cardiac event themselves, they're not in the "tribe." It's very easy for them to lose sight of the fact you're using humor to handle the emotional tensions heart disease causes and take the whole thing personally. You're supposed to be reducing stress. Fighting with your sweetheart is con-traindicated!

Risky Business (and the B.E.T. Method)

Sometimes humor just doesn't work. Have you ever told a joke or funny story and then have it fall flat? Sometimes it's the material itself that's not up to par; sometimes the audience ain't so swift; and some-times it flops because of its delivery. Sometimes trying to be funny can leave you with the taste of shoe leather on your tongue. Humor can be tricky!

There's a time and a place for everything, and that includes humor. You can minimize the risk of humor not working, and realize maximum benefits, by being mindful of where you are, who you're with, what they're likely to laugh about, and timing. I call this the B.E.T. method. (B stands for Bond; E stands for Environment; and T stands for Timing.)[1]

Humor: Here's how to make it a safe B.E.T.:

B = Bond

When we talk about Bond, we're talking about the relationship you have with the people you're about to share your humor with. Where are you connected? Are they family? What are their ages? Are they work colleagues? Are they neighbors (close neighbors vs. casual neighbors?) High school pals? Drinking buddies? Do you have a close relationship with the listeners, or are you not so sure of what will make them laugh?

Use some common sense here. Consider the people you're with at the time. Remember, other people won't change because you've had a heart attack! Their world view is likely exactly the same as it was before your cardiac event. If they're the type of people who get offended very easily, hold off on the questionable humor. On the other hand, if someone starts the conversation off with his or her favorite joke, you're probably safe using some humor of your own.

> **Re: Nature vs. Nurture: "Genetics loads the gun, and environment pulls the trigger."**
>
> **~ Dr. Francis Collins**

The longer you've known the person and the better the relationship is with them, the safer your humor will be. If you've previously shared some gross-out humor with your best friend, she may appreciate your joke that a porcine replacement heart valve will make you flinch at the sight of a porkchop. She may even laugh heartily. However, if it's someone you've known for only a short time, or have only known casually, you may want to mentally edit some of your humor before sharing it with him or her.

E = Environment

When we talk about Environment, we're talking about where you are when you're being funny. Being aware of the environment helps determine if humor is appropriate. Not all "clubs" are comedy clubs! For humor to be effective, you need your audience to be in a place where they're comfortable with humor. Some people don't joke in the workplace or in houses of worship, for example, but have no problem laughing it up in more casual settings. Not all types of humor work in all environments. The joke you tell while you're out at a bar might not be the same joke you tell during a family gathering. Now days, your environment might not even be physical—lots of humor is shared in cyberspace.

Anyone who hears your humor, sees your humor or experiences your humor is part of your audience, whether you meant for them to be or not. Maybe you're telling an off-color joke to your "Best Friend Forever" (BFF) at lunch but you tell it loud enough for the table behind you to hear—the family of four including two kids with big ears. Or maybe you send an email to a colleague with a sick joke in it and she posts it on her FaceBook page to her 1,317 followers (including your minister!)—still your audience.

T = Timing

You can have the right audience, in the right setting, and use humor—only to have it fall flat. Timing is perhaps the most difficult element to master when using humor. Have you ever heard people say, "Too soon!" to jokes about unfortunate events? They're not ready to laugh about the situation yet.

This can be particularly true if you're joking about your heart health. Other people, particularly the people who love us most, experience a significant emotional impact when we have a cardiac event. They're afraid, anxious, and overwhelmed too. Feeling forced to find the humor surrounding your heart health before they're really ready can provoke feelings of anger and frustration on their part.

How can you tell if the timing is right? How much time must elapse before an event can be funny? To be able to laugh at a moment or experience, you need to be able to emotionally detach from it. It has to be possible to look at the set of circumstances without re-experiencing the emotional response you had when the event occurred.

That process of detaching can take time. It's not an instant process—nor should it be! As complete human beings, we experience a range of emotions in response to life events. Anger, frustration, upset, and embarrassment have their role to play. These are life experiences that we learn from (eventually) and that help us grow.

After we've learned those lessons, it's time to laugh. Have you ever found yourself saying, "Someday I'm going to laugh about this"? At the peak of a crisis, nothing may be funny—but by recognizing that there is probably humor potential here that you'll be able to appreciate later, you're shortening the time frame between pain and play.

Some people can distance themselves immediately. They can laugh at their own mistakes—whether it's getting lost while driving somewhere, or saying something dumb in front of work colleagues. But other people need more time to process their reactions and emotions. When some people get lost, they berate themselves harshly. And as long as they are emotionally attached to the painful event, they will not find it funny. There are those who will just never see the situation as funny. That can be hard to accept, but it is as valid an emotional response as your decision to embrace humor.

Heart health involves practicing emotionally detaching from painful events, searching instead for the humor those moments contain. It isn't always easy, but with practice you'll find that you've developed the humor habit.

When to Use Humor?

Is it okay to laugh now??

Have you ever started to laugh, only to stop yourself? It can be difficult to gauge whether humor is appropriate or welcome in a given situation. Many times, we're so worried about whether laughing is really the right thing to do at any particular moment, that we censor ourselves, stopping ourselves from using humor.

I call this the "When in doubt, leave it out" approach. [You can also see this approach in my new cookbook, "Recipes with one ingredient or less!" Make sure to try the Strawberry Surprise!] The "When in doubt, leave it out" approach is, definitely, the safest option. You will never upset someone with the joke you didn't make. Use it too often, however, and you may leave yourself unable to capitalize on some of the many benefits of humor.

It's also important to remember to refrain from using humor during moments of crisis, or when it's vitally important that communication be clearly understood. Humor works by distracting the attention, and there are times when distraction is a very bad idea.

Lewis Grizzard, a heart patient, in his funny book, *They Tore Out My Heart and Stomped That Sucker Flat*, described his interaction with the nurse taking his medical history:

Nurse: "Pneumonia?"
Grizzard: "No."
Nurse: "Hemophilia?"
Grizzard: "Do what?"
Nurse: "Is there any history of hemophilia in your family?"
Grizzard: "Third cousin on my mother's side."
Nurse: "He was a hemophiliac?"
Grizzard: "Well, we weren't certain, but he wore ballet slippers to work."[2]

This humor worked because Grizzard's cousin wasn't actually a hemophiliac. Had there actually been a history of hemophilia in his family, this joke would have complicated the vital transmission of necessary humor. Talk about a sick joke!

Before using humor, do a quick check:
• What's my connection with the audience?
• Is this the right setting for this type of humor?
• Is this the right time to use humor?

The *Safest* Form of Humor

When in doubt about what kind of humor to use with others, use self-effacing humor (making fun of yourself). Sharing a funny story about yourself shows self-confidence and yet also shows vulnerability. People find this kind of humor totally non-threatening and may feel secure enough to share their own personal humor back with you.

Note 1: With self-effacing humor, it's best to focus on the funny or dumb thing that you *did*, and not position yourself as *being* dumb. Note 2: Using self-effacing humor requires self-confidence, and a strong sense of who you really are.

> *"I always wanted to be somebody,*
> *but I should have been more specific."*
>
> ~ Lily Tomlin

Remember this: You *are* somebody. Somebody who can be strong enough and confident enough to poke fun at yourself. Remember this, too: People who never use self-deprecating humor are not as confident and strong as they would like you to believe.

That's a little tidbit to keep in mind while using humor. Self-deprecating humor—the bit where you laugh at yourself—is a strong and powerful technique to help deal with chronic conditions, not to mention everyday life. The trick to self-deprecating humor is to make sure you focus on the things you *do*—and not the person you *are*.

Seriously. The world does enough to tear us down. We don't have to do it to ourselves.

"Laugh at your ACTIONS,
and not at WHO YOU ARE.
It's safer to admit you MADE a mistake
than to admit you ARE a mistake."

~ TERRY PAULSON, PH.D.

"Humor is power."

~ KARYN BUXMAN, NEUROHUMORIST

Chapter 4

You Want Me to Do *What?!*

—or—

Taking Action

So here we are. Now you know that humor has a ton of health benefits. Leveraging the power of laughter can have a tremendous positive impact on your physical and mental well-being. Let's talk about exactly how you can make that happen.

Heart disease changes everything. All of a sudden, you need to start eating better, exercising more, and stop stressing out—all of which is easier said than done! These changes impact you every single day. The most difficult part of any chronic condition is seldom the condition itself, it's the chronic part. Humor helps us cope as we navigate the many changes that come with heart disease, day-in and day-out. In this section, you'll find ways you can use the healing power of laughter to cope with heart disease.

> *"The most wasted day of all is that in which we have not laughed."*
>
> ~ NICHOLAS CHAMFORT

I've listed over two dozen ways for you to incorporate humor into your self-care. This is to give you a range of options. Think of this as the Grand Buffet of Humor. Take what you like and leave the rest! Don't feel obligated to pile everything onto your plate.

Humor is deeply personal. As you read through these pages, you'll find that some techniques and strategies make you laugh out loud, while others might not seem so funny. You'll realize maximum benefits by choosing and practicing those techniques and strategies that resonate with you. Choose the humor strategies that make you laugh, that you enjoy, and that seem far more like *play* than *work*.

I've divided the techniques into three main categories: Manipulating Your *Environment*, Manipulating Your *Mindset*, and Setting the *Pace*.

Life is Like a Dogsled Team (Manipulating Your *Environment*)

One of my favorite funny guys, Lewis Grizzard, had a great insight: "Life is like a dogsled team. If you're not the lead dog, the scenery never changes." Heart disease has a powerful way of making it clear: You're the person who has the most impact on what your life with heart disease is going to be like. Other people can certainly help pull the sled, providing love and support, but you're in the lead.

Being in the lead means you don't have to wait for someone else to step in and start making your life more fun. This is your opportunity to take action!

Incorporating humor into heart disease management means being proactive. There are simple steps you can take to cultivate the presence of humor in your life. Altering your physical surroundings can have a direct and dramatic influence on your mood. (Have you ever noticed how much better you feel immediately after walking out of the office? That's the power of altering your physical environment!)

There's a reason why people flock to the beautiful beaches of Hawaii for vacation. Simply being there can make you feel good. Realistically, few of us can afford to fly off to Hawaii every time we need a smile.

Luckily, there are easy ways to change your environment—and you don't have to worry about crowded airport security lines!

"Our bodies are helped to heal by engaging in those activities thaet bring us joy and fulfillment. Play is mandatory, it is not elective."

~ O. CARL SIMONTON, MD

The Power of Play

Here's what some of the exciting research from the world of psycho-neuro-immunology (PNI) tells us: Playful people are happier people.[1, 2] Happy people are healthier people. Play and humor are closely linked. One of the best ways to introduce humor into your day and more efficiently manage your heart disease is to embrace the power of play.

Playing, having fun, using the imagination—once upon a time, these were our only "jobs" in our lives. When we were kids, life was all about playing. Then, as the adult responsibilities began piling up, less and less time became available for playing. We've gotten too busy to have fun.

The *time* for play may have disappeared, but the

need for it has not. We still need our imagination, our silliness, our make-believe and clever games, as much as we did when we were kids. Perhaps even more, especially for Type A's who have had super-packed schedules that leave no time for fun. Play is incredibly powerful—it lifts the spirit, rejuvenates and energizes, and adds a much-needed element of joy to your day.

Play is so powerful and, almost universally, under-valued. Trust me, I've been paying attention (to children, to adults, to patients of many conditions, and to the medical and scientific journals). Play gets a bad rap, for being noisy, disruptive, and unproductive. For most of us, there's no place for play while we're on the clock—not if we want to keep our jobs!

Because children play, we consider play a childish thing—yet nothing could be further from the truth. Play can transform the way we see the world.

"I hated the wireless monitor," said Ronnie, a 56-year-old recovering from a triple bypass, "but the doctor wanted me wearing it. And then my grandson, Dylan, saw it. He thought it was the coolest thing—a remote control device for Grandpa!" Ronnie and Dylan played more than a few games of "Robot Grandpa." When Ronnie didn't need to wear the monitor anymore, he said with a grin, "I almost kind of missed it."

What Ronnie and Dylan had done was recognize and take advantage of the play potential hidden in what looked like ordinary home heart monitoring equipment. Kids can turn almost anything into a toy or game. Think about all the cardboard box forts and toilet paper tube kazoos that are out there! We can do the same thing as adults—and let's face it, now we have access to cooler stuff—and money!—with which to play "Let's pretend!"

Moving from the durable medical equipment arena, you can still play. If you want to incorporate more play into your life:

Create a Play List full of things that are fun for you![3] It can include games, playing with your kids or your dog [or your kids' dogs, or your dog's kids], skating, playing video games, etc. At least half the list should be low or no cost (unless you're both rich and have heart disease, in which case go wild—[and make sure your list includes, "Send large sums of money to my favorite humor author!"])

When it's been a bad day, or you're feeling down, do at least one thing on your Play List. There is a method to the madness here. When you're most in need of play is when you're least able to think of something fun to do. You're feeling sick or tired or frustrated—nothing sounds like much fun. And sometimes you're feeling like gum on the bottom of a shoe because your cash flow is so slow.

So do not wait until you feel better to do these things! Do them when you're feeling bad, and I promise, you will feel better.

"What if the Hokey-Pokey is really what it's all about?"

~ A BUMPER STICKER

Because really, is it even *possible* to have a bad day while dancing the Hokey-Pokey??

Build Your D-Team

Surround yourself with funny people! You want to build a team of positive people who enjoy life, like to laugh, and know how to have a good time. (I call this the D-Team, for the Delightful Team.)

This team has a critical role: To help you laugh more. Laughter is contagious. You can certainly enjoy humor when you're alone—but you're more likely to laugh and have fun when you're with others.

Research indicates that we're up to 30 times more likely to laugh with others than when we're alone.[4] (Who did this research? Great question! It was Sophie Scott, a neuroscientist at University College London, along with her colleagues.[5] [Hey, I really don't just make-up this stuff, you know!]) Our brains are wired to mimic the behavior we see exhibited by others; much the way you can acquire an accent when you travel far from home. When we see people laughing, we laugh too.

Capitalize on this tendency, and benefit from all the great things laughter can do for you, by creating and meeting with your D-Team on a regular basis. Taking in a funny movie, going to a comedy club, or simply getting together to hang out and have fun can all work.

> **Nearly 1 in 4 deaths in America are heart-related.** [8]

At the same time, your D-Team can serve as support and reinforcement for your own humor campaign. Think of your D-Team as external humor storage. They contain the funny that you may not have within you at a given point. Call them on bad days or when you're having trouble coping. Let them lift you up.

Support groups can be great places to meet people who are navigating the same challenges you are. Give yourself time to find the right group. You want to find a group of likeminded people who share a similar outlook on life. Each group has its own personality and dynamic. You want to find one that is a good fit for you.

"It was so funny. The very first support group I'd gone to, and I mean the very first one, was going along and a man announced that the woman who'd normally run the group wasn't there, and she wasn't going to be there, since she'd died in her sleep two days previous. And I'm sitting here thinking, 'This is going to lift me up? This is going to make me feel better?' Eventually I did find the right group of people, and it made all of the difference—but I'll never forget that first experience!" (Jill Knox, on finding the right support group.)

Being part of the D-team has benefits of its own. People who use humor regularly often find other people learn to depend upon them to brighten the day. This can create a strong positive expectation, giving you an impetus to look for humor in order to pass it along—which cheers you up in the process!

Handcuff the "Heart Attack Police"

Heart disease is astonishingly common. Experts tell us that at least 18 million Americans—that's one in every seven people—have been diagnosed with heart disease.[6] Even if someone doesn't have heart disease themselves, it's almost certain that they know someone who does. It may be a relative, a friend or a colleague. There's tons of information (and misinformation) floating around online and in the media about heart disease. Many people feel that they're pretty well informed about what it means to live a heart-healthy life—and once they find out you're dealing with heart disease, they feel compelled to share this wisdom with you!

Well-intentioned or not, it's time to admit that there's something fundamentally annoying about having a relative stranger watching every move you make as if you were about to suddenly clutch your chest and fall to the floor. It gets worse at the dinner table: Having your food choices scrutinized and policed by others is seriously annoying.

We have a name for those folks who think that your health condition gives them authority over your life choices: "The Heart Attack Police." They are attempting to control your behavior in order to prevent further cardiac complications. Their intentions may be good, but their approach is all wrong. In fact, the Heart Attack Police can increase the amount of stress in your life, rather than reducing it!

For that reason, it's more than okay to handcuff the Heart Attack Police. There are four ways you can do this. [Actually there are five, if you count shouting "FREEZE!" at the top of your lungs. This will work, but only momentarily.] You'll want to pick the way that's the most appropriate for the situation you're in (think back to that whole B.E.T. [Bond, Environment, Timing] section we covered earlier).

The goal is to minimize the negative impact that the Heart Attack Police have in your life, in a way that helps you preserve your energy and emotional resources. You want to be able to hold onto the positive aspects of your relationship with the Heart Attack Police. Remember, at some level, people engage in this type of policing behavior because they care about you. Giving them more appropriate ways to channel that concern is part of your self-care!

HOW to Handcuff the Heart Attack Police!

Option 1: Educate Them

Some people respond well to edification. Present the facts about your heart disease.

"My mother-in-law was freaking out about my plans to participate in a 1K Heart Walk," said Jenny R., who is diagnosed with atherosclerosis. "She didn't want me to do it, because she was scared what would happen. Finally, I had to tell her, 'Yes, I know I've got heart trouble. But the doctor said a moderate amount of exercise will actually do my heart more good than harm. I just have to know my limits.' That conversation helped her a lot, and she stopped trying to talk me out of going for my daily walk."

Option 2: Walk Away

You're not obligated to educate the world about heart disease. If someone is obnoxious, stubborn, or just not worth dealing with, walk away from the conversation.

"I guess there's one bad banana in every bunch," said Mark D., who's had two heart attacks. "Most of the people in our congregation are great, but there's one older gentleman who takes it really personally when I don't load down my plate at church suppers. I've tried telling him that the doctor has me on a strict diet—I don't want heart attack #3! But he won't listen. I've just stopped having that conversation with him anymore. It's not worth the headache."

Option 3: Get Your Expert On

Among all the people you know, who has more heart health knowledge than you? Let the Heart Attack Police know you're thrilled to discover they're really a cardiologist in disguise! This is your chance to get answers for your incredibly complex heart health questions—and you won't even have to pay a co-pay!

A note of caution: This method will not work on an inveterate 'truth-stretcher', the type who happily makes up answers as they go along. Exercise your judgment before implementing ANY of their suggestions!

Option 4: Disarm Them with Humor

"What do you mean the pig's valve doesn't come with a life-time supply of bacon?!"

Humor disrupts the conversation, disarms the Heart Attack Police's attempt to exert control over your life, and helps you maintain personal autonomy and dignity. The sneaky part is that you're not being critical or sharp, you're delivering your message with a smile and a chuckle. It helps to have funny quips and quotes to use on the Heart Attack Police. Deployed at the right time, these lines can turn a lecture into a laugh, and leave you both feeling better!

Here are some lines that have worked for folks I interviewed. Feel free to try these or come up with your own:

- *"Wow! Just eat healthy and exercise and my heart trouble will go away? That's **great**! It's a shame it hasn't worked for **your** little weight problem there."*

- *"Where were you when I was eating my salad? —Oh, so that was **you** over at the dessert table!"*

- *"Why yes, I **did** exercise. But I didn't see **you** in the gym this morning!"*

Be a Humor Collector

It's not always easy to find the funny. Some days are tougher than others. That's the nature of dealing with a chronic condition. You can be doing everything right—fabulous diet, exercising every day, swearing off the cigarettes, taking medicine as directed—and still have cholesterol numbers go sky high. There are days when everything hurts, no one understands you, and you are inexplicably without your flamethrower. [I would like to point out that I turned down a lucrative advertising opportunity from 'FlameThrowers R Us' to represent them, because that's how I roll.] Heart disease sends us on an emotional roller coaster. There are days when depression, anxiety, or plain old fear makes it hard to face the day.

Of course, those are the days when you need a laugh the most. These days happen to everyone. They're inevitable, because you're human. Lessen their impact by preparing yourself with a humor collection that you can access whenever you need it.

What goes into a humor collection? Well, comedians, obviously. Although you'll need a pretty large house in which to keep them all. [It has been brought to my attention since writing this book that some comedians object to being kept in people's personal collections, preferring instead to have lives of their own. Go figure! So please make sure to ask your comedian if he or she has any plans before adding them to your collection!] That's merely a starting point, though.

A complete humor collection includes:

Funny Movies

Films, TV shows, and even the occasional sporting event can produce genuine laugh-out-loud moments. (Remember way back when we were talking about all the research regarding humor? Many of the tests were run on people after they watched funny TV shows.)

Build a collection of your favorites—and remember, they don't have to be funny to everyone, they just need to be funny to you! [Not everyone appreciates the subtle comic genius of Gilligan.]

Netflix, Amazon Prime and other streaming video providers are great resources. [And with technology advancing at warp speed, you may soon be able to have "Cheers" downloaded directly into your brain!] You can watch funny films at anytime, anywhere. This is great if you live a long way from the movie theater or there's nothing on TV at 3 a.m. when you're wide-awake!

> **Q: What has the same physiological effects as losing 10 pounds? A: Participating in a "Laughter Group" for just 1 hour, every other week for three months.** [1]

YouTube is a treasure trove of funny videos. Create a favorites list of clips that make you laugh out loud for an instant pick-me-up. You can find humorous videos on virtually any topic. But just for you heart-oriented folks I discovered YouTube clips of David Letterman doing shtick about his quintuple bypass,[7, 8] Robin Williams doing stand-up about his heart valve replacement,[9] Regis Philbin joking about his bypass surgery,[11, 12] and Elizabeth Banks doing a wildly funny—and informative—bit on women and heart attacks (titled "Just a Little Heart Attack"). [13] Share your favorites with your friends. Humor shared is humor strengthened!

Funny in Print

Build a library of books that make you laugh. Sometimes books are funny because of the content, where other books are funny simply because they exist. *Even God Is Single, So Why Don't You Stop Giving Me A Hard Time?*, *Squee's Wonderful Big Giant Book of Unspeakable Horrors*, and *When Your Phone Doesn't Ring, It'll Be Me* are great examples—and you save money because you don't actually have to buy them; simply knowing about them makes you smile. (Yet another use for Amazon.com!) And Lewis Grizzard will have you laughing out loud with his book, *They Tore Out My Heart and Stomped That Sucker Flat!* Keep fun books on your shelf for easy access.

Don't feel limited to books, by the way: Magazines and newspapers can be great sources of humor. *Reader's Digest* is known for its humorous anecdotes. Most magazines have some sort of humorous column and many major newspapers carry comic pages. (When are the *Wall Street Journal* and the *New York Times* going to get a sense of humor, and add a comic section?) And you don't have to be a kid to buy a comic book! (Just ask the 140,000 people who attend Comic-Con every year—an annual event that everyone ought to experience at least once in their lives.)

Funny Art

There are all different kinds of art and some of it can be quite funny. The "Story People" art of Brian Andres can be humorous and profound, all at the same time.[14] Keep your eyes open and you'll start to see everything from stamp-sized funnies—remember the Bart Simpson stamps?—to yard-ornament-sized pieces of entertainment. A flock of pink flamingos can do wonders for your home's curb appeal.

> "The ability to laugh—either naturally or as a learned behavior—may have important implications in societies such as the U.S. where heart disease remains the number one killer. [6]
>
> ~ Dr. Michael Miller

Better yet, create your own fun art! There are countless art projects, shows and festivals with a heart health theme held across the nation every year. It's an amazingly short walk from a Heart Attack to an Art Attack, especially if you have a creative spirit. The very act of creating this art can boost your mood, lower your stress levels, and give you an outlet for your emotions.

Toys

You don't need to have kids to have toys in your house or office. Get some toys of your own! Maybe it's a Slinky, or a Rubik's Cube, or a Koosh Ball, or a talking stuffed heart (available in a rainbow of colors, including a very unhealthy-looking neon green)! Maybe it's a water gun or a stress ball that you can squeeze the heck out of. Ever play with Legos as a kid? You still can! (You can even 'connect' with other AFOLs [Adult Fans of Lego] at the annual BrickFair convention.) Your toy doesn't need to have any purpose other than to just bring a smile to your face when you play with it.

Cartoons

Cartoons, comics and other funny pictures can provide almost instant laughs and are yours for the clipping. But don't stop there! To get more mileage out of the cartoons, personalize them. Write in people's names or places of interest. Stick the cartoons on the fridge, tape them to your locker, mail them to a friend. Massage your creativity. White-Out the captions and come up with your own. *The New Yorker* magazine is well known for its cartoon caption contest (Don't get the magazine? You can still participate online.)

You might think that cartoons about heart disease would be hard to come by. But you'd be wrong! One of my favorite cartoonists, Johnny Hawkins, captures the funny side of healthcare in his *Medical Cartoon a Day* calendars. Available in e-reader format (get laughs right from your Kindle!) or in the traditional paper format, you'll have something to laugh at every day. And once again the Internet is a great resource—search for "heart health cartoons" and you'll find a variety of cartoonists to tickle your funny bone. Then take it another step: Try your hand at drawing some cartoons of your own.

Funny Audio

Listen to things that make you laugh! Collecting humor on CD or as a digital download makes it easy to get laughs any time you need them.

Commuters, this tip is for *you*! When traffic backs-up to a standstill and the guy behind you is laying on his horn, you can turn up the volume and laugh, instead of indulging in some free-form sign language. It's better for you and your blood pressure! [This tip is, of course, helpful for pedestrians, runners and couch potatoes, too!]

Here are some names to look for when you're googling for funny audio:

- Bill Cosby
- Steve Martin
- Robin Williams
- Tim Minchin
- George Carlin
- Lewis Black
- David Sedaris
- Daniel Tosh
- Jeanne Robertson
- Loretta LaRoche
- Tim Gard
- Karyn Buxman

Decorate for Laughs

Your living space has a huge impact on the way you view the world, yourself, and any place where the two interact. And by living space, I mean both your home and your workplace; after all, some of us spend more time at work than at home. [Type As, I'm looking at you!] That's part of the premise behind Feng Shui [the other premise being that if you let them, people will pay you large amounts of money to tell you how to arrange their furniture].

The same theories can be used to introduce elements of humor into your life. Altering your living space to make you laugh is simpler than you might think.

Embrace funny pictures and posters. Small figurines and knickknacks on a bookshelf can trigger a smile; seek out those objects that make you giggle and position them around your home.

At work, you can use your decorating efforts to inspire even more humor. Collect pictures of your colleagues and their pets—and see if people can pick out the pairs that go together. [Some people really *do* look like their dogs. Be prepared. You'll never look at a Basset Hound the same way again.]

As part of the lifestyle changes that come with a diagnosis of heart disease, you may find that you're spending more time in the kitchen. You're also spending more time in the room you work out in, whether that's the garage, family room, den or bedroom. Make these rooms enjoyable places in which to spend time! Introduce elements that make you smile. Hang a funny picture, stick some silly magnets on the fridge, replace your boring potholders with quirky mitts—the possibilities are endless.

Embrace Technology

No, this isn't all about your heart monitor! Through technology, we're all more connected than we've ever been before. The Internet, cell phones, social networking, you name it—the entire planet is no more than a click away. It's pretty amazing.

Why not harness this power to make you laugh? Start with your voicemail. Set it to leave a humorous message for all of your callers to hear. [You can do this with your personal voicemail and your professional voicemail. The professional voicemail can be a little tricky, so use your judgment. Not everyone wants to laugh when they call the funeral home, for example . . . so this might not be the best idea for morticians.] You'll be amazed at how many jokes you'll get

> *YouTube could save a friend's life: Send her to "Just a little heart attack."*

in return [particularly if you're really subtle and say something like, "Leave your name, number, and favorite joke!"]. You'll laugh when you listen—and you're sharing the joy.

Use RSS readers or news aggregator programs to collect all of your favorite funny blogs and websites into one convenient location. You can read these on your smart phone, tablet, or computer. It's an easy way to get a daily dose of funny without having to go looking for it: A real time saver! (Don't have favorite funny websites or blogs yet? Give yourself a gift and take an hour or two to explore the Internet. Google "Heart Disease + Humor + Blog" and you'll be amazed at what you'll find. Of course you don't have to limit your search to heart health-related material, but it's a good starting point, and there's great value to be found in having an online community.)

There are numerous sites that will deliver the joke-of-the-day (or the cartoon-of-the-day, the cat-photo-and-funny-caption of the day, the funny-horoscope-of-the-day—you get the picture) directly to your email or cell phone. Sign up for one. That way you have a guarantee each and every day that there will be something to laugh about—and you don't even have to remember to hunt for it—it will be right there on your computer or phone.

Our enjoyment of humor increases when we share it with others. We're social creatures, which is a huge part of the reason social networking has become so popular. Check-out Facebook, Twitter, and a gazillion other sites. Use your social networks to share and solicit humor. Posting a joke to a wall only takes a minute, and seeing the responses gives you an added boost. [Even if they're just Likes or smiley faces!] Ask for jokes and links to funny material—people love to share humor!

YouTube

- America's Funniest Home Videos
- Bloopers from your favorite TV shows
- Bloopers from your favorite films
- Classic comedy, from Laurel and Hardy to Abbott and Costello to Burns and Allen
- Dr. Demento
- Just a little heart attack
- David Letterman heart attack
- Robin Williams heart attack
- Laughing babies
- Funny cats

Other Funny Stuff Online

- www.FunnyOrDie.com
- www.CollegeHumor.com
- www.VideoBash.com
- www.TheOnion.com
- Google "funny quotations"
- Google "Garrison Keillor"
- Google "Ellen DeGeneres"
- Jib Jab eGreeting Cards
- eGreeting Cards featuring Hoops & Yoyo
- Google "funny stuff"
- Google "humor"
- Google "humorists"
- Google "comedians"
- Google "funny songs"
- Google "Monty Python"
- Google "Laugh In"
- Rubber Chicken eCards

Apps

On a *serious* note . . . Here are some apps that, while they ain't funny, just might save your life!

- WebMD: Health info and tips
- iMuscle: An "anywhere" workout
- Calorie Counter: For diet and activities
- Nike Training Club: Your own "personal trainer"
- The Eatery: Improve your heating habits
- Fooducate: Scans product barcodes
- P90X: A workout that tracks your performance
- Fitness Class: Video workouts
- Gorilla Workout: Fitness training on a budget
- Medscape: Medical news and education
- Dining Out Guide: Make healthy food choices

Bring Humor to Your Doctor

Heart disease changes the environment we live in. Our regular routine expands to include trips to the doctor, cardiac rehab center, the pharmacy, and other medical facilities. It's more of a change than most people realize at first. Learning what your life will be like after a cardiac event takes time and energy. There's a significant time commitment involved. That's part of the reason why managing heart disease often feels like another full time job on top of the ones you already have!

Introducing some humor into the process makes it easier to deal with. Bear in mind that this is something you're going to have to initiate. The same healthcare professionals who won't hesitate to crack a chest are very wary of cracking jokes—unless you do it first. Once you've demonstrated that you're open to and enjoy humor, they're much more likely to give you something to laugh about.

> **The major risk factors for heart disease:[5]**
> **Inactivity**
> **Obesity**
> **High blood pressure**
> **Cigarette smoking**
> **High cholesterol**
> **Diabetes**

Humorist Lenny Dave tells how he used humor while waiting for his angiogram. "The morning was filled with numerous tests on some truly amazing pieces of equipment. One test was basically a cardiac sonogram, not unlike when they "looked" at my then-pregnant wife's belly. They rubbed this blue goo on my chest and pressed a magic gizmo against it. As I lay there, I could see the monitor. I just had to know, so I asked the technician, "Can you tell? Is it a boy or a girl? Does it have a little 'thingy'?"

Knowing that humor is a tool both you and your healthcare providers can access makes some of the more difficult conversations easier. Heart disease is not an easy thing for anyone. No one likes being confronted with his or her mortality. It's scary to face up to the fact that there are parts of our lives that are beyond our control. There are few moments as terrifying as those when you realize you can't predict what happens next. Often, we spend these terrifying moments in the company of our healthcare providers. Doctors, nurses, and cardiac rehab professionals are there as our lives change before our very eyes. When we use humor, it gives our medical support team the permission to use humor to help us.

Lenny Dave tells what happened during his angioplasty. "As I lay on the operating table awaiting the 'happy juice' to start flowing into my IV, I tilted my head to look over at the skilled, cardiac surgeon whom I really had met only briefly up in the Emergency Room. He was all prepped in his sterile gown, rubber gloves and what looked like an OSHA-approved welder's mask. Now, I knew full well that this guy had probably performed this procedure thousands of times. But, with a semi-straight face, I inquired, "So Doc, have you EVER done one of these things before?"

With perfect vaudevillian timing and without missing a beat, he said, "Well, I tried it yesterday on the dog!"

A Note About Timing

Bringing humor into a medical setting is fine—much of the time. However, if you or someone nearby is in a crisis situation, humor can be inappropriate and distracting, and take the focus away from where it needs to be. Use your best judgment.

Party ... Just Because

Hallmark has it right: Life is a special occasion! Take the time to celebrate. Birthdays and holidays are great opportunities to get together with family and friends for a great time—but there's no reason to limit yourself to these occasions. Increase the amount of humor and fun by throwing parties . . . just because.

Create events or festivities "just because." Theme days are a great idea (such as Beach Day, 70s Day, Country Western Day, etc.) where you focus on doing something fun that is tied to the theme. The Beach Day could include a Gidget movie marathon; a Country Western Day could include songs that never made the big time ["You're The Reason Our Kids Are So Ugly" or "Get Your Tongue Outta My Mouth 'Cause I'm Kissing You Goodbye"]; and we don't really want to know what you're going to wear on 70s Day!

This doesn't have to be a great big deal to deliver great big results. Just try integrating the theme into your everyday activity: Bloggers could post about the theme, inviting readers to share their stories. You could dress in the appropriate attire. Dare to be a little bit silly, just for the joy of laughing and making others laugh.

Theme days offer the opportunity to have a gathering that isn't necessarily about food. This cuts the Heart Attack Police off at the knees—unlike most of our holidays which are celebrated with the ABC's (Alcohol, Baked Goods and Chocolate)—when it's your celebration, you can set the menu! [It would be, perhaps, cynical to suggest a fantastically healthy menu containing no salt, fat or flavor whatsoever. Everyone else should love it, since they recommend it so heartily (pun intended) to you!]

These ideas work best when you have buy-in from your family, friends, or co-workers. If you're in a supervisory capacity, encourage your entire team to get involved: This boosts morale as well as your own spirits.

Change the Scenery

Managing heart disease is, in large part, all about establishing new routines. Eating healthier meals and taking the time to smell the flowers is only the beginning. Add to that the daily medication, regular workouts at the gym, and routine doctor's appointments and you can find yourself in a rut before you know it.

That's why it is essential to shake up the day and introduce elements of spontaneity and delight into your day. For some folks, it's the daily routine of heart disease management that becomes a drag. These tasks everyday can wear on your soul. If that's the case, you'll want to change things up.

The easiest way to do this, of course, is to give your car keys or cell phone to a nearby toddler, and tell the rugrat to put them somewhere safe for you. The sheer challenge of trying to find out where that may be, using only your approximation of toddler logic and acrobatic skills, can shake up your morning for hours at a time. [And don't try to take the easy way out and ask the toddler where your keys are. Not because it's not sporting, but because—honestly??—they're not going to remember!!]

If you're not quite that open to adventure [also known technically by the pros as "sane"], you can still introduce some elements of serendipity and surprise into your day. Commit to trying something fun and new each week: Read a new blog; go to a new restaurant, a new activity or class. Take a new route on your daily walk. Listen to a different style radio station than you usually do. Sleep on the opposite side of the bed than is your habit [you may want to give your partner the heads-up on your experiment, first!].

"Novelty is the parent of pleasure." [Robert South said this. I'm not sure who he is, but in case you wanted to know, there you go. William Thackeray, on the other hand, whom I *was* previously aware of, said, "Novelty has charms that our mind can hardly withstand," which is a good quote too.] Provide yourself with a regular diet of new experiences and you will find yourself having more fun!

If I Hadn't Believed It...
(Manipulating Your *Mindset*)

Congratulations! You've learned how to increase the amount of humor in your life by manipulating the environment. Now it's time to talk about how the way you *think* about your life impacts your heart disease. Using simple tools and techniques, you can develop a humorous perspective that makes facing down the daily challenges of heart disease much easier. What a gift! The ability to tap into humor whenever and wherever you want to means you've got a totally portable skill set to use whenever you need it.

Raise Your Awareness

If you want more humor in your life, you have to look for it. I call this raising awareness. Raising awareness means choosing to recognize the funny side of life and deliberately cultivating laughter and mirth in your life.

Raising awareness means choosing to ask questions like, "What's so funny about heart disease?" There's a reason I titled this book with that curious phrase. It's a good question. Heart disease is a serious, life-altering condition. What's there to laugh about?

Heart disease, in and of itself, is not particularly funny. I've examined the medical literature from every angle, and there's just not anything inherently humorous about it.

Living with heart disease, however, is another story—and that's really what we're talking about here, isn't it? *You are more than your diagnosis.* You are not defined by whether you've had a bypass—or a double, or triple, or a quadruple, or even a quintuple! Your pacemaker is not more important than your personality. Heart disease is just a part of your life, not the entirety of it, and the rest of life is actually pretty funny.

OVERHEARD IN THE OR:

"I don't think my wife likes me very much.
When I had my heart attack,
she wrote for an ambulance!"

Sometimes that humor is dark. "How do you manage the stress of heart disease with everything else that goes on in your life?" a patient on an online heart health forum asked. Only a few moments elapsed before the first funny answer was posted. "Interpretive dance and sky diving! Works for me!" [Obviously, your mileage may vary. Interpretive dance just isn't for everyone!]

The first step in using humor to help manage your heart disease is coming to peace with the fact that while heart disease *isn't* funny, the challenges that come along with it sometimes *are.* Dark humor, sarcastic humor, clever wordplay, slapstick comedy, good practical jokes, bubbly friends, puns that will make you groan, and everything in-between can help you feel better.

Sometimes we have weird cultural baggage about our health. We're often taught that certain topics are "Off Limits"—too serious, too delicate, too impolite, too personal, too important, too critical to laugh about. What can be more serious than a heart attack? It doesn't seem right to laugh about the health changes that have disrupted our lives. But now, it turns out that it's time to let that go. Your health depends on it. Understanding the role that humor can play in heart health management makes letting go of "Off Limits" easier. Practice helps too. [And that's how you get to Carnegie Hall!]

Don't worry—the practice is actually quite fun. We'll be getting to that next.

Seek to Find the Funny

It's a lot easier to SEE funny than to BE funny, and it's more valuable, too. Seeing funny is one of the easiest ways to integrate humor into your life. In fact, once you start, you might not be able to stop!

"If I hadn't believed it, I wouldn't have seen it."

~ ASHLEIGH BRILLIANT

The very first step in seeing funny is to assume that there's funny to be seen. If your worldview tells you, "There's nothing funny happening in my life," then you'll be right. On the other hand, if you believe that the world is an amusing place just waiting for you to discover it, then you'll be right, too.

Let yourself believe that the world is full of humor. Just taking this simple step will place you light years ahead of those around you who are in too much of a hurry to take a moment to see and hear and experience the vast absurdity and delight going on all around us.

This can be hard for some folks, especially if you're a fairly tightly wound Type A. If this is you—if you're certain that the world is continually on the edge of disaster that can only be avoided if you, yourself, personally manage everything and everyone—you've got permission to start with baby steps. Don't try to see everything that's funny around you. Just look for one or two things every day, things that you can laugh about easily and without effort. You'll find it gets easier as you practice.

The search for funny is really changing the way you view the world around you. In a way, you're cultivating a deliberate mindset—a lens through which you view the world, opening yourself up to a funny interpretation of everyday sights, sounds, and events.

Look for funny signs. My personal current favorite is the New Mexico road sign that promises:

> ABSOLUTELY NOTHING
> NEXT 12 MILES

Newspapers, magazines, television—especially local news broadcasts—and websites produce tons of inadvertent bloopers that can provoke a smile.

Here are some actual newspaper headlines that will bring a smile to your face. (Sometimes the humor is on purpose; and sometimes it's humorously unintentional!)

> CITY UNSURE WHY SEWER SMELLS

> ONE ARMED MAN APPLAUDS
> KINDNESS OF STRANGERS

> PUMPKIN PRODUCTION PATCHY

> SOMETHING WENT WRONG IN JET CRASH,
> EXPERTS SAY

> HOW TO BUY A $450,000 HOUSE
> FOR ONLY $750,000!

Listen for the funny things people say. Kids, friends, celebrities, politicians—they're all funny. Sometimes it's even on purpose! Check out the countless quote books and numerous websites devoted to the amazing things people say. For instance:

"You have to stay in shape.
My grandmother started walking five miles a day
when she was 60. She's 97 today,
and we don't know where the hell she is!"
~ ELLEN DEGENERES

"Always go to other people's funerals,
otherwise they won't come to yours."
~ YOGI BERRA

"The best cure for insomnia is to get a lot of sleep."
~ W.C. FIELDS

There are literally hundreds of thousands of funny quotes out there, from people famous, infamous, and unknown. For a simple way to add humor to your life, make a practice of finding one funny quote or anecdote each and every day. Write it down, post it on Facebook, or share it with the family over dinner,

Creating a "humor journal" is another good idea. Knowing you need to record something—anything—every day, can help you train yourself to recognize and appreciate the funny moments that are all around you.

The items in your humor journal don't have to be magnificently funny, although sometimes they will be. For example, one morning at a busy grocery store, I watched a harried woman with an overflowing cart just crammed full of groceries cut to the head of the Express Lane—"10 Items Max." (Apparently 27 cans of cat food only count as one item in some people's minds.) She was a bit curt with the cashier, explaining that she was in a hurry.

The cashier, not missing a beat smiled sweetly and said, "No problem! Which ten items would you like to buy?" [Don't you just LOVE it!]

One technique to remind you to look for the funny is to put a small dot with marker, pen, makeup, etc. on your wrist. Any time you notice it throughout the day, stop, look around, and take note of what's humorous around you right that minute.

Celebrate Your Achievements

You are an amazing person, and you do amazing things! Make a point of celebrating your personal achievements. Don't wait for people to give you the recognition you deserve. Practice enthusiastic standing ovations for yourself.

You brought your cholesterol down 30 points? Whoop it up and celebrate! Give yourself three solid minutes of applause!

Stuck to your new diet—even though there were some beautiful double-bacon-cheeseburgers available at the company BBQ? That calls for the Woo-Hoo Dance of Triumph!

Stopped the Heart Attack Police cold in their tracks? Nothing will do but an NFL-style end-zone celebration, complete with spiking a football. This is particularly amusing if your run-in with the Heart Attack Police happens at work. [But if you happen to actually *be* an NFL player, don't do this. It'll cost you a boatload of money for misconduct.]

Let's be serious for a moment and look at why this works. Positive reinforcement, boiled down to its essence, is the concept that "The behavior that is rewarded is the behavior that is repeated." [This was stolen from my buddy Rick Segel, co-author of *Laugh and Get Rich*. Don't tell him!]

It doesn't matter, technically, who does the rewarding. What matters is that you get the recognition and appreciation for the positive things you do to manage your heart disease. That means it's more likely that you'll continue to practice these positive behaviors. You're creating the change you want in your life. That's worth celebrating.

No one is closer to your heart disease than you are. That means that try though they might, no one on this planet is as aware of your triumphs and achievements as you are—not your partner, not your parents, not your healthcare provider, not your best friend. Nobody knows you as well as you do. You are the person perfectly positioned to provide this positive reinforcement. *You* are the Number One choice to be your own cheerleader!

Of course, once you start the celebration, there's nothing to stop your friends from joining in. Fun shared is fun amplified—the more the merrier! (When you become aware of your friend's triumphs and accomplishments, celebrate them! It makes both of you feel good and allows you to benefit from the healing aspects of humor even more.)

Give Yourself Permission to Laugh Alone

Humor is among the most intimate and personal of emotions. What makes us laugh is highly individual and unique. I've heard it said that senses of humor are like fingerprints: No two are alike. What's funny to you may not be funny to someone else. Have you ever found yourself laughing hysterically at something only to have one of your coworkers look at you disdainfully and say, "*That's* not funny"?

Now here's a story that generates a variety of reactions from people:

"This joke always gets me into trouble," said Simon, a 57 year-old steelworker with cardiomyopathy. "But I'll tell it to you anyway: Fred played golf every Sunday. One Sunday he came home from the golf course much later than usual.

"Bad day?" his wife asked.

"It started out great. Two birdies on the front nine!" he said. "Then Harry had a heart attack and died on the 10th tee."

"Oh, that's awful!"

"You're not kidding. For the whole back nine it was hit the ball, drag Harry, hit the ball, drag Harry."

Some folks laugh right out loud when they hear Simon's joke. Others find it cold, uncaring, and just not funny. What matters, though, is that *Simon* finds the joke funny—every time he tells it, he laughs until he cries.

This may happen to you. It's hard to predict what will tickle your funny bone. What happens when you're the only person laughing? It can certainly feel awkward. It helps to say, "You know, I'm my own best audience. And I just do this for my own amusement." Yes, humor can be used to entertain and lift the spirits of those around you, but it's also effective and appropriate to use humor to make yourself feel better.

Think of it as self-care. It's not hurting anyone, and it's benefiting you. If you stop and think about it, very little of your self-care actually requires buy-in or participation from other people. Do you have an audience every time you get on the treadmill and log another mile? Do you take your meds on camera so everyone can enjoy the moment? Do you have a cheering squad every time you have oatmeal for breakfast instead of a stack of sausages? [If you do, could you send the squad to me? I've somehow misplaced mine!] Don't worry if other people "don't get it"—they don't have to for it to make you feel better.

Actively Embrace Humor as Part of Your Treatment Regime

The best thing you can do to manage your heart disease is work closely with your doctor, cardiac rehab team, and support system to make positive changes in your life. Their advice is life-saving. So implement those changes!

Luckily, you don't have to limit yourself to one tactic or technique to help you manage your heart disease. You've got the freedom and flexibility to do what you think is best to boost your heart health. Humor has a huge role to play here—and it's not likely to be included in the advice from most healthcare professionals—at least not yet. But we know that humor complements everything you're already doing!

A small warning for you: While I do advise you to become more conscious of your humor, don't over-analyze it. A curious phenomenon that those of us in the "humor industry" have noticed is that the more you analyze humor, the less funny it becomes. This is especially pertinent for you Type A's who consider analysis their favorite sport!

"Humor can be dissected as a frog can, but the thing dies in the process, and the innards are of interest to only the pure scientist."

~ E.B. WHITE

Of course, phrases like "consciously choosing to make humor part of your treatment plan" sound suspiciously like serious business. Most of us never think about what makes us laugh, or why, from an analytical point of view. It can be a little intimidating.

Intimidating, that is, until you realize the vast number of laughs that are derived from pictures of cute animals with witty captions (thank you, www.icanhascheezburger.com), physical mishaps (*America's*

Funniest Videos, anyone?), and the foibles of society's "beautiful people" (this is the entire reason for *E! News'* existence). This is not particularly sophisticated material here—nor does it have to be.

What we're talking about is the process of identifying what makes you laugh. What does it take to amuse you? Where's your sure source of smiles? Pinpoint what

More than 616,000 Americans died of heart disease in 2008. [8]

tickles your funny bone, and start taking steps to make that a regular part of your life. Humor is essential. You want to have it in your routine, right along with eating right and the daily workout. Consider your time laughing and playing as much a part of your heart health management as watching your cholesterol and stress control.

Who says you can't enjoy something that's good for you? Think about it: The next time you're on the couch, laughing at your favorite comedy, you're actually doing something to manage your heart disease!

A side note: If your significant other suggests that helping clean the garage is also a great way to help your heart health, it might be wise to listen to him or her! The cardiovascular benefits aside, you get to skip the fireworks when you say, "I just have to see the end of *Dumb & Dumber*, honey!"

Humor is a fantastic heart disease management tool. It's completely portable and always available. You can laugh anywhere, anytime. No equipment is required, and it doesn't cost any money. Humor is there when you're tired, scared, stressed out or fed up!

Prop Yourself Up

There's a reason comedians and magicians use props: They're fabulous for provoking laughs. One easy way to up the amount of humor in your life is to stock up on funny props. Tuck a clown nose in your desk drawer, Groucho glasses in your glove box, and a magic wand near the microwave. The magic wand comes in particularly handy when you're confronted with a surly teenager who's gotten off of his cell phone long enough to stare sullenly into the refrigerator and share his first words in two days with you: "There's never anything to eat around here!" This is the perfect time to use that magic wand to make him disappear. Magical moments mean family memories!

Having funny props readily available makes it easy to get people laughing—and chances are you'll be joining right in. Simply slipping on a pair of Groucho glasses can transform your morning commute—try it and see!

Psychologist Steve Sultanoff, a professor at Pepperdine University, is a master of using props in everyday life to lighten the mood and connect with others through humor. (HumorMatters.com) Ask him what time it is and you'll see that his watch runs backwards [reading *that* takes talent—and/or a twisted mind!]. Ask for his identification and you'll see versions including John Wayne, Marilyn Monroe or Elvis! He's quick to don a red clown nose— great for getting a reaction at fast–food drive-thru's. In December he wears a button that that has a capital L with a slash through it. It takes most people a few moments before they decipher the "secret" Christmas message: "No L"—"Noel" . . . get it?! He notes that not only does it make him feel better, but that there is a ripple effect. Others appreciate his humor and want to pay it forward.

> "The old saying that 'laughter is the best medicine' definitely appears to be true when it comes to protecting your heart."[6]
>
> ~ Dr. Michael Miller

Having funny props around can bring a smile to your face, simply by the virtue of their presence. One of my favorite people, Fran London—creator of *The*

Laughing Buddha, and former editor of the *Journal of Nursing Jocularity*—talks eloquently about the value of funny props. She says, "There's something very powerful about having a collection of tangible items that make you laugh." Harness this power with your own personal collection of bobble-head dolls, rubber chickens, or whatever makes you smile!

There are two types of props. *Universally* humorous props are those that make everybody [okay, *almost* everybody] laugh. You have here your helicopter beanies, giant clown shoes, and oversized sunglasses. *Personal* props are those items you keep on hand because they make *you* laugh. These don't necessarily have to be funny to anyone else. [Not everyone appreciates the comedic potential of Chia Pets; and no one else needs to know why that picture of Elvis cracks you up.] Mix and match until you find the right balance for you.

Let the Music Move You

They say that music can soothe even the most savage beast. I'm not sure that's true—taking on lions, tigers and bears armed only with *Celine Dion's Greatest*

Hits might be more than a little dangerous! But what we *do* know is that music is a powerful tool that can lift the mood, elevate spirits and positively impact your emotional state. Your personal playlist can be a tremendous asset in helping you manage your heart disease.

The trick to using music to regulate your mood is to find music that's personally relevant to you. That's actually a little easier for people with heart disease. Sometimes it seems like you can't turn on the radio without hearing something that'll inspire greater heart health:

Achy Breaky Heart—Billy Ray Cyrus
Don't Go Breaking My Heart—Elton John
How Can You Mend a Broken Heart?—Bee Gees
Every Beat of Your Heart—Rod Stewart

When all else fails, fall back on old favorites. See if you can recall the theme songs to *The Addams Family* or *The Beverly Hillbillies*. Try out your favorite Christmas carols. *Grandma Got Run Over By a Reindeer* works really well for this, particularly in July.

Expand Your Definition of Intimacy

Yes, we're going to talk about *that*. [In an all-ages, family-friendly-type of language. Otherwise, I'd be able to charge a lot more for this book!] Heart disease can have a tremendous impact on one's sex life, for reasons both physical and emotional. This can be a problem, as the connections we have with our partner are a critically important part of our lives. In fact, some people argue that this is the *most* important part of life. [Personally, I'd put my local comedy club in first place, but you'll have to take this up with my husband, who has agreed to put up with my quirkiness.]

When problems occur, we have two options. The tried and true do-absolutely-nothing-about-it-hoping-the-problems-will-just-magically-resolve-of-their-own-accord strategy is very popular. It somehow persists despite the fact that it doesn't work at all.

The second option, which I talked about with Dr. Ed Dunkelblau, the Director of the Institute for Emotionally Intelligent Learning, involves using humor and rethinking your definition of intimacy.

For many people, the definition of intimacy and the definition of sex are one and the same. Expanding the definition of intimacy to include more than sexual intercourse will benefit every couple, not only those couples that include a heart patient. This means exploring different kinds of touch, closeness, and the conversations one has with one's partner.

"Intimacy can be defined as the exchange of vulnerabilities," Dr. Dunkelblau said. "Which means it's critically important that the humor you share be positive humor." Positive or constructive humor is laughing *with* someone, not *at* someone. Bear in mind that we all have a fear of being judged or

> "*Nonsense makes the heart grow fonder.*"
>
> ~ Karyn Buxman
> neurohumorist

rejected in intimate situations; it is essential that we don't poke fun nor use mean spirited sarcastic humor during these times. [And here's a tip for the ladies: When in bed, never, never, *never* point-and-laugh at the same time.]

"Anxiety is at the root of many difficulties," Dr. Dunkelblau explained. "Humor reduces that anxiety, which has obvious physical effects. It's not unheard of for couples to find that time together, sharing laughter, can then lead them back to a space without that anxiety, to a place that is more enjoyable."

It's important to remember that no one is alone in facing this challenge: There are now increasing numbers of resources available, with specific tips and techniques to enhance intimacy while managing a chronic condition. Explore what works for you, and don't forget the value a good laugh can add.

Here are some specific resources for you:
- www.Heart.org
- www.GoRedForWomen.org
- www.FrankTalk.org
- www.InvisibleDisabilities.com
- www.WebMD.com
- www.WhatsSoFunnyAbout.com

Set the Tone for Conversations

If you manage the message, you'll manage the day. When someone asks you how you're doing, don't just answer, "Fine." Enthusiastically answer, "*Incredible!*" and watch the startled smiles appear.

One of the most draining aspects of managing heart disease (and pretty much any other chronic disease)—is people's unwanted questions and advice. "Why can't someone ever just say, "What's up?" asks George T. "Instead every conversation turns into an interrogation about my health."

Even if you've got good news to report, it doesn't take long to feel like your heart condition dominates your conversation. This makes it difficult to maintain the positive, upbeat attitude we're aiming for. It clouds that lens we talked about earlier, the one you use to find the humor in the world.

But you have control over the types of conversations you have and the messages you put out there. Answering "*Incredible!*" when someone asks how you're doing is a great way. You're "derailing" the conversation by providing someone with an answer they didn't expect—and the answer is lighthearted and upbeat, which is often a different tone than what is expected.

You can also take control of the message by limiting how many times you're going to explain your health situation on any given day. Make an agreement with those near and dear to you that unless you say otherwise, they can assume that all is well on the health front. After all, you don't inquire daily about their cholesterol levels, migraines, and that embarrassing boil on their butt. [If you have people who just won't get with the program, make a point of asking them intimate details about their health on a daily basis. Preferably in front of other people. When they protest, innocently say, "I'm just *concerned* about you . . ."]

Don't minimize your condition when things are going badly, but on the other hand, don't dwell on the small stuff when things are actually going pretty well. You'll find you get more meaningful responses and concern when this type of conversation is limited—and more joy when the alternative is funny stuff!

Catastrophize It!

You're on your way to your cardiac rehab appointment and you're stuck in traffic because some kind soul decided to text while driving [obviously not the sharpest knife in the drawer], accidentally ran into a fire hydrant, and has now flooded your route with water and stalled cars. Yep, you're going to be late all right.

Ever have one of those days? Sometimes it's the small stuff that makes us sweat; the miniature aggravations that throw off our equilibrium. It's tempting to minimize the impact of the steady stream of seemingly small incidents that distress, dismay, and discombobulate ["Now THERE'S a funny word."] us—until, that is, we remember that it just takes one more straw to break the camel's back, one last grain of sand to empty the hourglass, one additional drop of water to fill the cup to overflowing and send waves of negative emotions and wild behavior everywhere. We cannot ignore these small things. Individually, they aren't much, but collectively, they are everything.

The trick is to keep things in their proper perspective. One technique to stop the small moments from accumulating into an unmanageable mass is "Catastrophizing." [Sometimes the name of this technique causes confusion. Rest assured, it has absolutely nothing to do with contributing to the ranks of male sopranos.]

Catastrophizing is a game you can play by yourself. When you're confronted with an issue that's relatively minor, ask yourself, "How could this be worse?" Each answer should mirthfully exaggerate the situation.

To wit: "Well, I could have been on my way to the airport instead of rehab . . . and missed my flight to the Bahamas . . . and been stranded in traffic for DAYS . . . with a car full of obnoxious relatives... one who has a tiny bladder... another who's gassy... and another in active labor!"

Ridiculous? Of course. But at some point, you're going to laugh [or at least smile]. And you're going to remember that you're freaking out over a common, everyday traffic back-up. And from there, you can move on.

Practice Humor Visualization

It's always best if you can surround yourself with people who make you feel great, who make you laugh and who enjoy your company, as well. But let's face it. Sometimes you're stuck with a person who is driving you nuts. What's a person to do? Practice the art of Humor Visualization, or the art of playing with your comic mindset. No one is going to know just what pictures you've conjured up in your head—unless you're laughing so hard that you give it all away.

> *Humor helps some people reduce their bad cholesterol (LDL) while increasing their good cholesterol (HDL).* [2]

For instance, you love your job, but there's that guy in the next cubicle who has driven many a former employee to drink [White-Out, that is!] with his annoying habits. The next time he begins ranting that the coffee is too cold, try picturing him tipping over backwards in his chair—with his expensive tie drenched with coffee—along with his computer, which is shorting-out! [Now THAT'S funny.]

What would your CEO look like wearing clown pants, a curly rainbow wig and a red rubber nose? Could you imagine the most annoying customer in the world doing a Lady Gaga impression? The possibilities are endless.

Take a Mental Trip

This is somewhat similar to the previous exercise, in that it involves picturing something amusing in your mind. But in this case, you're going to tap into fun and pleasant memories. We all have the classic stories we tell to family or friends when we get together and reminisce. Like the time Aunt Clarice (5 feet tall and 5 feet wide) fell on her back in the snow and flailed like a turtle on its back, screaming for Uncle Carl to come flip her over [you had to be there]. Or how your brother snuck the car out on the Fourth of July only to have a sack of fireworks in the back seat get set off by a stray bottle rocket that flew through an open window and eventually burned out the interior of the entire car after a dazzling display lasting over 20 minutes [true story—just ask my brother!].

The trick is to start purposefully collecting a repertoire of these stories and tapping into them. It wouldn't hurt to write down a list at first. Then periodically, take a moment to think back to these moments of mirth. Your body can't tell the difference between a *real* humorous event in the moment or an *imagined* event that is being recollected from the past. Both are going to do great things for your body chemistry.

Be Grateful

Gratitude is a powerful emotion. It's almost as powerful as humor, and when you combine the two, you can really benefit. So the trick is to find funny things about heart disease to be grateful for.

I realize this can be kind of tricky, so I'll give you a few of my favorites to get you started.

- Because you've followed your diet so well, you can now fit into the same clothes you wore in college [remember that plaid leisure suit?!].
- Your health insurance plan covers you even better than your hospital gown did.
- Your in-depth, up-close and personal relation ship with heart disease allows you to speak with authority on the subject, and throw around polysyllabic words like they were confetti. [If, however, you're at a wedding, opt for the confetti. It's a rare bride indeed who enjoys her nuptials being showered with poly-syllabic words.]

You can be grateful in how you *act*, and also in how you *think*: Many folks find a grateful mindset through prayer or meditation.

Laugh at Yourself

"You grow up the day you have your first real laugh — at yourself."

~ ETHEL BARRYMORE

When all is said and done, you should take your heart disease seriously—it's serious stuff. But you can take *yourself* lightly. Learn to separate the two. *You are not your disease.* You are an amazing and amusing individual with a rich resource of life experiences. You just happen to have a cardiovascular disease.

Hopefully with the tools and information I've given you, you can put yourself and your life in their proper perspective. Laugh at your mistakes, your foibles, and your embarrassing moments, as well as your successes, your pleasures, and your joy-filled moments. Life really is too short to take it so darn seriously!

What are You Waiting For?!
(Setting the *Pace)*

Start Your Day with Laughter

Mornings are hard. Is there anything harder than getting out of bed, especially if you know that's going to be followed by the morning trip to cardiac rehab? ["Especially when the route to rehab fails to include major attractions, like Dunkin' Donuts or Starbucks!"]

Behavioral researchers have found that the beginning of our day tends to set the tone for the remainder of that day. My friend, Dr. Robert Holden, of The Happiness Project, recommends that we ask ourselves, upon waking, "How happy do I choose to be today?"[2]

You would think everyone would automatically say, "I choose to be super happy!" But that's not usually the case. Most of us have a 'range of happy' we're comfortable with: It takes exceptional events to make us happier than we normally are.

You can adjust those settings and expand your range of happy. One way to do this is to incorporate humor into your morning routine. Make sure you have something to laugh about in the morning.

This may reveal the underutilized value of humorous coffee mugs. [I received no financial support from the Humorous Coffee Mug Association to say this. However, if they would like to send me some cash as appreciation for this recognition, I'll be glad to accept it. You could also buy me off with a bunch of mugs—I'm clumsy, and could always use replacements.] Sign up for a joke-of-the-day email that's delivered first thing in the morning. Find a drive-time radio show that makes you laugh. If you can't find anything amusing, fake it.

Experts have discovered that even fake laughter has benefits. [Not the least of which is that participating in laughter clubs and laughter yoga stands you a better than fair chance of showing up on local media, particularly during the slower periods of the news cycle.]

> *From my favorite coffee mug:*
> *"I don't have a short attention span, I just . . .*
> *Oh, look! A squirrel!"*

Several years ago, Charles Schaefer, a psychology professor at Fairleigh Dickinson University—and co-founder of the International Association for Play Therapy—conducted a study that demonstrated that even completely fake laughter can boost mood and overall well-being. In the study, participants were asked to laugh heartily for one full minute. Afterward, they reported feeling better, with a more positive outlook on life. The study was repeated with similar results, and has formed the basis of many laughter groups.[15]

Laughter clubs can be found in many locations, particularly if you live near a large city. These can be a great resource, offering a chance to connect with other like-minded individuals. You can find out more by visiting www.WorldLaughterTour.com to find existing groups or to learn about forming your own laughter club.

Here are some laughter exercises you can try [and these will all work in the privacy of your own home, if you're more comfortable doing this where no one can see you!]:

Flying Bird Laughter

Swoop around the room, flapping your arms like the wings of a bird, laughing all the while. Change the type of bird: Are you a slow moving albatross, gliding over the ocean, or a fast flying hungry eagle zooming to your next meal?

Electric Shock Laughter

Pretend you're getting an electric shock from everything you touch. Give a great big exaggerated response to every pretend shock: Jump up in the air, wave your arms, yell "Aye Carumba!" and laugh.

Hula Hoop Laughter

Imagine a Hula Hoop around your hips. Get the hoop moving by swinging your hips in a circular direction—and laugh while you keep the hoop in motion.

Hearty Laughter

Laugh while raising both arms toward the sky with your head tilted a little bit backwards. Feel as if the laughter is coming from your heart. [Frankly, at first, I thought this exercise was silly. But I tried it—and now it's my *favorite!*]

Gradient Laughter

Start by smiling—then slowly begin to laugh with a gentle chuckle. Increase the intensity of the laughter until you've achieved a hearty laugh. Then gradually bring the laughter back down to a smile again. [I wonder if it's normal to break into maniacal laughter, like 'Bwaa-ha-ha-ha!'?]

Schedule a Humor Break

Make time for humor every day. This can be the five minutes in the morning that you spend reading jokes online or the half hour you spend watching an episode of your favorite sitcom at the end of the day.

Anticipating fun can have nearly as many positive benefits as actually experiencing it. [There has been extensive research on this phenomenon, particularly by the Thursday-Sneak-Out-of-the-Office-and-Catch-a-Matinee-While-Everyone-Thinks-You're-at-a-Big-Important-Meeting Club.] For this reason, you'll want to load your calendar with fun events you're looking forward to. Movies, time with friends, an evening at a comedy club—don't view these things as indulgences; consider them a critical aspect of creating a healthy lifestyle. [Alas, not so critical that your insurance company will pay for them; good luck submitting a movie stub for reimbursement!]

Develop humorous traditions. If you know that the third weekend in March will always be your comedy movie marathon, where you gather with all of your friends and spend the weekend laughing, that weekend takes on a special significance and meaning to you. It also strengthens bonds and builds community: People who can never find a spare six seconds in their schedule tend to find the time to have a good time, particularly when they can plan for it in advance.

Planning for humor doesn't reduce the chances of spontaneous laughs happening throughout the day. If anything, giving yourself deliberate opportunities to recognize and enjoy humor actually prepares you to appreciate the funny moments in life when they crop up on their own. You're training yourself in a new way of viewing the world: Look for the funny, and you will find it.

On Your Mark, Get Set . . .

Go! What are you waiting for? There's no time like the present to get started and begin putting humor into your life starting right now! *When humor happens by chance you get some **benefits**—but when you begin using humor **proactively** you will create some **amazing, life-changing results**.*

Check back in and let me know how it's working for you. I want to hear your experiences. And I'm always looking for a good story or joke. [Did you hear the one about…?]

"Warning: Humor may be hazardous to your illness."

~ ELLIE KATZ

Chapter 5

The Last Laugh

David Letterman—a healthy and avid runner—felt a pressure in his chest. Four hours later he was undergoing quintuple bybass surgery.

Robin Williams—a healthy, energetic guy (albiet with a fondness for cocaine)—experienced a sharp pain in his chest during a live comedy performance. The next day an angiogram confirmed the diagnosis: The very funny man had had a very serious heart attack.

Barbara Walters—a woman with no history of heart disease in her family, who popped out of bed at 5 o'clock every morning and took a brisk walk, who had never missed a day of work in her life—felt a pressure in her chest while strolling through Central Park. Two months later she had open heart surgery.

Regis Philbin—the Energizer Bunny of talk shows and game shows—announced during a 2007 episode of *Live with Regis and Kelly* that he would be undergoing triple bypass surgery later that week, as he had recently experienced chest pains and shortness of breath.

Rosie O'Donnell—known for her humor and outrageousness (but not for her good health!)—felt nauseous and clammy one night. She thought, "Nah! This isn't a heart attack!" but took an aspirin just in case. She waited a day before checking into a hospital—where she discovered that her coronary artery was 99 percent blocked.

Bill Clinton—who ran 20 miles per week (interspersed, of course, with greasy hamburgers)—experienced . . . well, you know what happened!

* * *

Fame, money and power will not protect you from heart disease. It happens to the best of us. It happens to those who exercise. And to those who don't. It happens when you least expect it. *And* . . . it is not necessarily a death sentence. It can be the beginning of a whole new life. And it just might be the best thing that's ever happened to you! (*If* you take its lessons to heart.)

* * *

Every one of the six people profiled above recovered quickly, and returned to their work and their lives with a newfound vigor and enthusiasm. And, every one of them made lifestyle changes based on the latest recommendations of the American Heart Association. *And*, every one of them used their influence and their media platforms to share their experiences and educate the public about the importance of heart health.

David Letterman—following a two-month hiatus from his *Late Night* TV show—returned to the stage accompanied by two nurses; he was greeted by a standing ovation that lasted a full minute; he leaned into the camera and began his monologue with these words, "You won't *believe* what happened to me!" He then proceeded to entertain and educate his millions of fans, using his heart attack as the launching-point for the humor *and* the education. (Note: And while Letterman was recovering, his friend Regis Philbin, though a "morning person," substituted for the *Late Night* host.

Robin Williams—when deciding on whether to get a bovine heart valve, or a pig's heart valve, or a mechanical heart valve—asked his doctor if he could get "the new Apple iHeart"! His advice to people considering open heart surgery: "You want the surgeon who's performed *thousands* of operations. You don't want the doctor who's only done, like, *six*!" Williams used his heart attack experience in his subsequent comedy shows. "You come out the other side, and you're okay, and it's '*You* Two-Point-Oh!' You've got another chance at life! I don't want to just 'smell the roses'—I want to smell *all* the flowers!"

> "Humor by CHANCE can be beneficial, but humor by CHOICE creates amazing, life-changing results."
>
> ~ Karyn Buxman, neurohumorist

Barbara Walters—discussing her operation during a TV special on heart disease—said, "It's no big deal—just a matter of life-and-death!" When her physician said that she had about one year to live if she did not have an operation, she said, "Open heart surgery? Me?!" She was so surprised and skeptical that she got a second opinion—and then a third, and then a fourth! And then—she went in for the operation. Three months later she was back on *The View*, interviewing President Obama (the first sitting American president to appear on a TV talk show).

Regis—who underwent triple bypass surgery—joked with his medical team the day after his surgery.

And while he was recovering, his friend David Letterman returned the favor and co-hosted Regis's show until he recovered.

Rosie O'Donnell—who says that a TV commercial about heart health saved her life—urges women not to discount the warning signs as she initially did. In her blog she wrote: "Know the symptoms, ladies. Listen to the voice inside. The one we all so easily ignore."

Bill Clinton—following his emergency bypass procedure—changed his eating habits and became a vegan. When he appeared on the *Late Night Show*, David Letterman asked him, "I've been struggling with *my* weight—and you've conquered *your* weight! What are you doing, how you doing it, and why-can't-I-do-it?!" Mr. Clinton answered, "Well, I gave up meat, dairy and fish. And I eat as close to a vegan diet as I can get." Letterman responded, "*Wow!* —Well, see, I don't want to do *that!!*"

* * *

Different people, different paths. Same outcome: Renewed health and vigor.

What's *your* path?

* * *

So here we are, at the end of the book. I hope you enjoyed reading this half as much as I enjoyed writing it [which was a *lot!*]. It's more enjoyable than working out on the treadmill, anyway . . . right? And packed with nearly as many benefits!

Adding humor to your healthy-heart-management kit is painless, and should be a lot of fun. Remember that the benefits of humor increase when they're shared. And besides, laughing with someone else is fun in-and-of-itself!

Take time every day to treat yourself well. You eat healthy every day [okay, every day that is *not* Halloween], you exercise every day—[don't go there]—all for the sake of a healthy heart. It's time to add *one more* element: Enjoy humor every day. (This isn't just good advice based on anecdotal evidence. It's scientific fact based on solid neurological research. [See the footnotes for references to articles published in peer-reviewed journals.][1])

My neuroscientist friends are proving that there are causal links between humor and health, humor and happiness, humor and creativity, humor and success, and humor and life balance.

Laugh often, laugh deeply, laugh with others, and laugh alone. Laugh in the morning and laugh in the evening. Laugh knowing that you're reducing stress, improving your health, and most importantly of all, that you're having fun.

Humor is as crucial as monitoring your meds, as critical as getting your exercise, and as joyful as discovering a heart-healthy version of your favorite childhood treat.

Here's one last joke, just to leave you laughing . . .

"My doctor told me to avoid stressful situations . . .
so I didn't open his bill."

[Ha!]

4 out of 5 doctors recommend*

(Online resources can deepen your understanding of applied and therapeutic humor, and of heart health.)

Association for Applied & Therapeutic Humor
www.aath.org

This non-profit organization serves as the community for professionals who study, practice and promote healthy humor. (Non-professionals love it, too.) Services include a monthly ezine, teleconferences, an annual conference, CEs, and graduate credit available through the Humor Academy.

American Heart Association, www.Heart.org

The official site for the American Heart Association providing articles, resources, news, research and much more.

Comic-Con, www.Comic-Con.org

An annual gathering of 140,000 fans of popular culture, including movie fans, sci-fi fans, Star Wars aficionados, super hero lovers, and comic book fans. Loads of programs and products sure to make you laugh!

---

* Dr. Seuss, Dr. Kildare, Dr. Hawkeye Pierce, Dr. Who

Go Red for Women
www.GoRedForWomen.com

A passionate, emotional, social initiative designed to empower women to take charge of their heart health.

Invisible Disabilities Association
www.InvisibleDisabilities.com

A non-profit organization providing education, encouragement and community to anyone who is touched (whether directly or though a loved one) by a disability that may not be physically obvious. They're raising awareness and helping decrease the stigma of having an invisible disability, including chronic pain, chemical sensitivities, or post-traumatic stress.

Laughter Yoga, www.LaughterYoga.com

Founded by Dr. Madan Kataria, Laughter Yoga combines unconditional laughter with yogic breathing (Pranayama). Exercises, events, and information available.

The New Yorker Cartoon Caption Contest
www.NewYorker.com/humor/caption

A weekly contest where anyone can submit captions to a cartoon provided by *The New Yorker*. The winners' captions appear in the magazine. No cash prizes, but it's great for bragging rights!

StoryPeople, www.StoryPeople.com

Unique and playful illustrations, artwork, physical and electronic greeting cards and more, with funny and/or insightful thoughts by artist Brian Andreas.

WebMD, www.WebMD.com.

Great articles and resources on heart health.

What's So Funny About® . . .?
www.WhatsSoFunnyAbout.com

Neurohumorist Karyn Buxman's blog on using applied and therapeutic humor in your life. Topics focus on specific conditions/diseases (diabetes, cancer, depression, Alzheimer's, heart disease, etc.), and on specific professions/roles (nurses, caregivers, leaders, business, relationships, parenting, etc.).

World Laughter Tour,
www.WorldLaughterTour.com

Founded by Steve Wilson and Karyn Buxman to support, promote, and act as a clearinghouse for the global laughter movement, with the mission of bringing events to every continent that supports health and peace through laughter. Articles, exercises, events and news.

(Ruptured) Appendix

Sidebars

1.
Peeples, L. (March 28, 2011). Laughter, Music May Lower Blood Pressure. Retrieved from: http://www.cnn.com/2011/HEALTH/03/25/laughter.music.lower.blood.pressure/index.html

2.
Lee Berk, PhD; Earl Henslin, PsyD., MFT, BCETS; Steve Sultanoff PhD; & Kathleen Passanisi, PT, CSP, CPAE; April 8, 2011 presentation, "Science Fiction, Science Fact, or What We Just Want to Be True," Association for Applied & Therapeutic Humor annual conference, Anaheim CA.

3.
Roger VL, Go AS, Lloyd-Jones DM, et al. Heart disease and stroke statistics—2012 update: a report from the American Heart Association. Circulation. Epub 2011 Dec 15.

4.
Heidenreich PA, Trogdon JG, Khavjou OA, et al. Forecasting the future of cardiovascular disease in the United States: a policy statement from the American Heart Association. Circulation. 2011;123:933-44. Epub 2011 Jan 24.

5.
National Center for Health Statistics. Health, United States, 2010: With Special Feature on Death and Dying. Hyattsville, MD.

6.

University of Maryland Medical Center. (April 24, 2012) Heart Disease: Tips for Prevention. Retrieved from http://www.umm.edu/features/tips_prev.htm#5

7.

Barbara Walters. "A Matter of Life and Death," TV special. ABCNews, February 4, 2011.

8.

Miniño AM, Murphy SL, Xu J, Kochanek KD. Deaths: Final data for 2008. National Vital Statistics Reports; vol 59 no 10. Hyattsville, MD: National Center for Health Statistics. 2011.

Chapter 1

1.

National Heart Lung Blood Institute. (March 1, 2011) What is a heart attack? Retrieved from http://www.nhlbi.nih.gov/health/health-topics/topics/heartattack/

2.

Roger, V., Go, A., Lloyd-Jones, D., Benjamin, E., Berry, J., Borden, W., Bravata, D., Dai, S., Ford, E., Fox, C., Fullerton, H., Gillespie, C., Hailpern, S., Heit, J., Howard, V., Kissela, B., Kittner, S., Lackland, D., Lichtman, J., Lisabeth, L., Makuc, D., Marcus, G., Marelli, A., Matchar, D., Moy, C., Mozaffarian, D., Mussolino, M., Nichol, G., Paynter, N., Soliman, E., Sorlie, P., Sotoodehnia, N., Turan, T., Virani, S., Wong, N., Woo, D. & B. Turner, M. (December 15, 2011) Heart Disease and Stroke Statistics□□2012 Update A Report From the American Heart Association: Circulation Retrieved from http://circ.ahajournals.org/content/early/2011/12/15/CIR.0b013e31823ac046.citation

3.
Miniño A., Murphy S., Xu J, & Kochanek KD. (2011) Deaths: Final data for 2008. National Vital Statistics Reports; vol 59 no 10. Hyattsville, MD: National Center for Health Statistics.

4.
McNair, T. (February 2009) Heart attack recovery. BBC Health. Retrieved from http://www.bbc.co.uk/health/physical_ health/ conditions/in_depth/heart/heartattackrecovery1.shtml

5.
Maddox, T. (June 28, 2012) Edema overview. Retrieved from http://www.webmd.com/heart-disease/heart-failure/edema-overview

6.
Beckerman, J. (February 16, 2012) Symptoms of heart disease. Retrieved from
http://www.webmd.com/heart-disease/guide/heart-disease-symptoms

7.
Mayo Clinic. (January 12, 2011) Heart disease. Retrieved from http://www.mayoclinic.com/health/heart-disease/DS01120/DSEC-TION=symptoms

8.
Health Net Federal Services. (nd) Heart failure education. Retrieved from: https://www.hnfs.com/content/hnfs/home/tn/bene/wellness/ dis-ease_managementinformationcenter/heart_failure_education.html

9.
Jefferson, A., Himali, J., Beiser, A., Au, R., Massaro, J., Seshadri, S., Gona, P., Salton, C., DeCarli, C., O'Donell, C., Benjamin, E., Wolf, P., & Manning, W. (2010). Cardiac Index Is Associated With Brain Aging: The Framingham Heart Study. Circulation, 122, 690-697.

Chapter 2

1.
Saturday Night Live. (nd) Season 3, episode 18, Theodoric of York Medieval Barber. Retrieved from: http://www.hulu.com/watch/3529/saturday-night-live-theodoric-of-york

2.
Buxman, K. (1990). The professional nurse's role in developing a humor room in a health care setting. Masters Thesis, University of Missouri, Columbia.

3.
University of Maryland Medical Center. (April 24, 2012) Heart Disease: Tips for Prevention. Retrieved from
http://www.umm.edu/features/tips_prev.htm#5

4.
American Heart Association. (February 27, 2012) Cardiovascular Disease and Diabetes. Retrieved from
http://www.heart.org/HEARTORG/Conditions/Diabetes/WhyDiabetesMatters/Cardiovascular-Disease-Diabetes_UCM_313865_Article.jsp

5.
Lee Berk, PhD; Earl Henslin, PsyD., MFT, BCETS; Steve Sultanoff PhD; & Kathleen Passanisi, PT, CSP, CPAE; April 8, 2011 presentation, "Science Fiction, Science Fact, or What We Just Want to Be True," Association for Applied & Therapeutic Humor annual conference, Anaheim CA.

6.
Robinson, V. (1991). Humor and the health professions. Second Edition. Thorofare: Slack Publications.

7.
Berk, L.; Tan, L.; & Tan, S. (2009). Mirthful laughter, as an adjunct therapy in diabetic care, increases HDL cholesterol and attenuates catecholamines, inflammatory cytokines, C-RP, and myocardial infarction occurrence. FASEB Journal, 22, 1226.2.

8.
Berk, L.; Tan, S.; Fry, W.; Napier, B.; Lee, J.; Hubbard, R.; Lewis, J.; & Eby, W. (1989). Neuroendocrine and stress hormone changes during mirthful laughter. American Journal of Medical Science.298(6), 390-396.

9.
Peeples, L. (March 28, 2011). Laughter, Music May Lower Blood Pressure. Retrieved from
http://www.cnn.com/2011/HEALTH/03/25/laughter.music.lower.blood.pressure/index.html

10.
Fry, W. (1979). Humor and the human cardiovascular system. In H. Mindess, J. Turek (Eds.). The study of humor. Los Angeles: Antioch University.

11.
Fry, W. (1992). The physiological effects of humor, mirth, and laughter. Journal of the American Medical Association, 267 (13), 1857-1858.

12.
Park, A. (February 29, 2012) FDA Warns Statin Users of Memory Loss and Diabetes Risk. Retrieved from
http://healthland.time.com/2012/02/29/fda-warns-statin-users-of-memory-loss-and-diabetes-risks/

13.
Hayashi, K.; Hayahsi, T.; Iwanaga, S.; Kawai, K.; Ishii, H.; Shoji, S.
& Murikami, K. (2003). Laughter lowered the increase in post-prandial
blood glucose. Diabetes Care, 26 (5), 1651-1652.

14.
Hayashi, T. & Murakami, K. (2009). The effects of laughter on post-
prandial glucose levels and gene expression in type 2 diabetic
patients. Life Science, 85(5-6): 185-187.

15.
Berk, L.; Tan, L.; & Tan, S. (2009). Mirthful laughter, as an adjunct
therapy in diabetic care, increases HDL cholesterol and attenuates catecholamines, inflammatory cytokines, C-RP, and myocardial infarction
occurrence. The FASEB Journal, 22, 1226.2.

16.
Seiler, B., & Levitt, B. (March 9, 2009). University of Maryland School
of Medicine Study Shows Laughter Helps Blood Vessels Function Better.
Retrieved from http://www.umm.edu/news/releases/laughter2.htm

17.
Ohio State University Medical Center. (nd) Retrieved from
https://patienteducation.osumc.edu/Documents/distrhum.pdf
18.
Galloway, G. & Cropley, A. (1999). Benefits of humor for mental health:
Empirical findings and directions for further research. Humor 12-3,
301-314.

19.
McGhee, P. (2010). Humor. The lighter path to resilience and health,
pp. 96-101. Bloomington, IN: AuthorHouse.

20.
Goldstein, J. (1987). Therapeutic effects of laughter. In W.F. Fry &
W.A. Salameh (Eds.), Handbook of humor and psychotherapy. Sarasota,
FL: Professional Resource Exchange.

21.
Grizzard, L. (2010). They tore out my heart and stomped that sucker
flat. Montgomery, AL: NorthSouth Books.

22.
Wilson, S. (nd), The World Laughter Tour and laughter therapy.
Retrieved from
http://www.worldlaughtertour.com/sections/about/difference.asp

23.
Provine, R. (2000). Laughter: A scientific investigation. NY: Penguin.

24.
Cousins, N. (1984). The healing heart. NY: Bantam.

Chapter 3

1.
Buxman, K. (1998). Humor as a cost-effective means of stress management. Managing Employee Health Benefits, 6 (2), 74-78.

2.
Grizzard, L. (2010). They tore out my heart and stomped that sucker
flat. Montgomery, AL: NorthSouth Books.

Chapter 4

1.
Seligman, M. (2004). Learned optimism. How to change your mind and your life. NY: Random House.

2.
Holden, R. (2010). Be happy! Release the power of happiness in you. Carlsbad, CA: Hay House

3.
O. Carl Simonton, presentation at The Laughter and Play Conference, Clearwater FL, November 1989.

4.
Griffin, R. (nd). Why We Laugh. Retrieved from
http://men.webmd.com/features/why-we-laugh

5.
YouTube. (June 29, 2012). How We Learn to Laugh- Professor Sophie Scott (UCL) Retrieved from : http://www.youtube.com/watch?v=wD3TcORDs3I

6.
Heart Disease and Stroke Statistics; 2012 Update: A Report From the American Heart Association: Roger, V., Go, A., Lloyd-Jones, D., Benjamin, E., Berry, J., Borden, W., Bravata, D., Dai, S., Ford, E., Fox, C., Fullerton, H., Gillespie, C., Hailpern, S., Heit, J., Howard, V., Kissela, B., Kittner, S., Lackland, D., Lichtman, J., Lisabeth, L., Makuc, D., Marcus, G., Marelli, A., Matchar, D., Moy, C., Mozaffarian, D., Mussolino, M., Nichol, G., Paynter, N., Soliman, E., Sorlie, P., Sotoodehnia, N., Turan, T., Virani, S., Wong, N., Woo, D. & B. Turner, M.
Circulation published online December 15, 2011
http://circ.ahajournals.org/content/early/2011/12/15/CIR.0b013e31823ac046.citation

7.
YouTube. (March 12, 2007). David Letterman Jokes about Heart Surgery. Retrieved from
http://www.youtube.com/watch?v=KhFkC1Z18c8

8.
YouTube. (January 19, 2008).Late Show with David Letterman- Heart Surgery 8th Anniversary. Retrieved from
http://www.youtube.com/watch?v=N1oNCgzfbOc

9.
YouTube. (November 17, 2011) Robin Williams Talks about Heart Surgery. Retrieved from http://www.youtube.com/watch?v= PkO8zsScsa4

11.
YouTube. (April 26, 2007). Heart Bypass with Regis and Letterman- Part 1. Retrieved from http://www.youtube.com/watch?v=dwNHKtginec
12) YouTube. (April 26, 2007). Heart Bypass with Regis and Letterman- Part 2. http://www.youtube.com/watch?v=mFnTfMgEiXl

13.
YouTube. (August 31, 2011). Go Red for Women presents: Just a Little Heart Attack. Retrieved from
http://www.youtube.com/watch?v=t7wmPWTnDbE

14.
Andreas, B. (1997). Story people: Selected stories and drawings by Brian Andres. Berkely, CA: West Coast Print Center.

15.
Schaefer, C. "Laughter," FDU Magazine Online, Winter/Spring 2006. Retrieved from
http://www.fdu.edu/newspubs/magazine/06ws/laugh.html

Chapter 5

1.
"Therapeutic Effects of Forceful Goosing on Major Affective Illness";
Copans, Stuart A.; Journal of Irreproducible Results, 1985, Dorset
Press. [The Journal of Irreproducible Results is a forum for the humorous, satirical, and critique writings concerning those in whom the hallmark of achievement has resulted in jargon, pomposity, verbosity and
obfuscation to befuddle the uninitiated and preserve the mystique that
often clothes the culprit or the ignorant.] Really. You could look it up.

A special thanks to my contributors

Lenny Dave, Founder and President of Lenmar Communications, is a nationally recognized speaker, humorist, creative thinker and author. He is Past President of the Association for Applied & Therapeutic Humor (AATH). Lenny is also co-founder of the National Collegiate Speakers Association. Over the past 25 years, Lenny has addressed a variety of audiences of all ages around the country. *Campus Activities Magazine* has twice nominated Lenny as "Speaker of the Year." Lenny is co-author of "Let Your Leadership Speak: How to Lead and Be Heard" and "Choose Courage Over Fear: Decisions That Determine Your Destiny."

www.LennyDave.com

Ed Dunkelblau, Ph.D., is a licensed clinical psychologist and nationally known speaker on the topics of social-emotional intelligence, humor, and health. Dr. Dunkelblau has two master's degrees from Columbia University: one in psychology and the other in vocational and rehabilitation counseling, and a Ph.D. in counseling psychology from the University of Kansas, where he was recently recognized as a distinguished alumnus. He has been in clinical practice for 25 years, is Past President of the Association for Applied & Therapeutic Humor (AATH), is approved supervisor for the Association for Marriage and Family Therapy, and director of the Institute for Emotionally Intelligent Learning.

www.teacheq.com

Steven M. Sultanoff, Ph.D., is a psychologist, university professor (Pepperdine), professional speaker, and internationally recognized expert on therapeutic humor. With over 25 years in the therapeutic humor field, he is the author of many innovative articles, and his chapter "Integrating Humor into Psychotherapy" appears in *Play Therapy with Adults*. Dr. Sultanoff has appeared on *The Morning Show, Lifetime, STARZ,* and PBS and is frequently interviewed and quoted in national publications. He is Past President of the Association for Applied & Therapeutic Humor (AATH) and has been awarded the AATH 2012 Lifetime Achievement Award. His highly ranked (Google) web site (humormatters.com) provides a wealth of information on therapeutic humor.

www.HumorMatters.com

Index

Books by Karyn Buxman, RN

What's So Funny About . . . Diabetes?

What's So Funny About . . . Heart Disease?

What's So Funny About . . . OR Nursing?

What's So Funny About . . . School Nursing?

Amazed & Amused

Laughing Your Way to More Money, Better Sex & Thinner Thighs

Humor Me (co-author)

The Service Prescription (co-author)

Chicken Soup for the Nurses Soul (contributor)

Coming soon in the "What's So Funny About...®?" series

What's So Funny About . . . Alzheimer's?

What's So Funny About . . . Cancer?

What's So Funny About . . . Depression?

What's So Funny About . . . Parkinson's?

What's So Funny About . . . Aging?

What's So Funny About . . . Dialysis?

What's So Funny About . . . Love?

Karyn Buxman, RN, MSN, CSP, CPAE

The Really Important Stuff

Karyn Buxman is an RN with attitude . . . and a serious sense of humor. As a nurse, she cared for hundreds of patients one-on-one; as a motivational keynoter, she now administers to thousands of people from the stage. Karyn is a neurohumorist—one who researches the neurobiology and psychology of humor, and then translates cutting-edge findings for the layperson, showing how they can harness applied humor to heal and empower themselves.

Karyn presents laughter with a purpose. Mirth with a message. Humor that heals. Keynotes that enlighten, educate and entertain. Karyn's key messages include "Humor is power," and "It is more important to *see* funny, than to *be* funny." Karyn has been described as "One part Norman Cousins, one part Patch Adams, and two parts Lucille Ball."

The Additional Stuff

But wait—there's more! . . . There's that mind-body-spirit connection thing! As a researcher *and* performer, Karyn brings science, psychology and humor together with health, success and spirituality.

What else? . . . Karyn has addressed 5,000 members of the Million Dollar Roundtable in Thailand; rocked 8,500 OR nurses in Chicago; and presented her research at the International Society for Humor Studies in Paris. (Oh! She's also addressed the US Air Force, Pfizer, the Mayo Clinic, and 1,197 other organizations.)

Karyn has authored six books, she is published in peer-reviewed journals, and she is an inductee into the Speaker Hall of Fame (one of only 37 women in the world). She is a contributor to two *Chicken Soup* books, and she is the author of the *What's So Funny About...?* series *(WSFA...Diabetes? WSFA...Heart Disease? WSFA...Nursing?)* She was given the Lifetime Achievement Award from the Association for Applied & Therapeutic Humor. Karyn's mission in life is to improve global health through laughter, and to heal the humor impaired.

858-603-3133   KARYNBUXMAN.COM